Facial Gua Sha

Text by Zhang Xiuqin
Translation by Shelly Bryant
Cover Design by Shi Hanlin
Interior Design by Wang Wei

Assistant Editor: Yang Wenjing
Editor: Cao Yue

ISBN: 978-1-63288-017-8

Address any comments about *Facial Gua Sha* to:

SCPG
401 Broadway, Ste.1000
New York, NY 10013
USA

or

Shanghai Press and Publishing Development Co., Ltd.
Floor 5, No. 390 Fuzhou Road, Shanghai, China (200001)
Email: sppd@sppdbook.com

Printed in China by Shanghai Donnelley Printing Co., Ltd.

1   3   5   7   9   10   8   6   4   2

The material in this book is provided for informational purposes only and is not intended as medical advice. The information contained in this book should not be used to diagnose or treat any illness, disorder, disease or health problem. Always consult your physician or health care provider before beginning any treatment of any illness, disorder or injury. Use of this book, advice, and information contained in this book is at the sole choice and risk of the reader.

Facial Gua Sha

A Step-by-Step Guide to Achieve Natural Beauty through **Traditional Chinese Medicine**

By Zhang Xiuqin

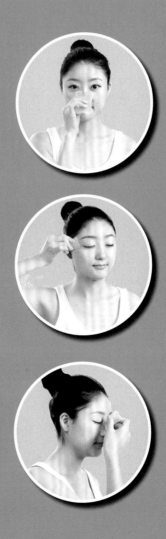

SCPG

CONTENTS

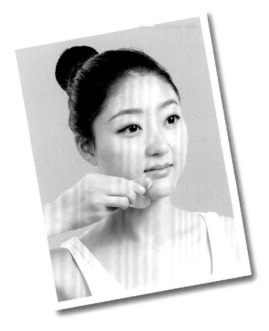

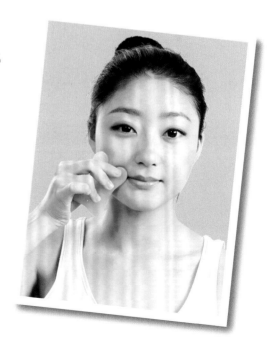

FOREWORD

As time goes by, our faces take on the imprint of the years, recording old scars and fresher emotional wounds. Wrinkles, spots, and acne on the face are not only unsightly; they are also a sign that something is wrong inside our bodies. Solving these problems requires a comprehensive adjustment from the inside out.

Since the launch of my holographic meridian facial *gua sha* method, many people have vouched for its beautifying effects, but I also discovered two major misunderstandings about *gua sha*: the first is that not everyone masters the essentials of facial *gua sha*, often confusing it with techniques for body *gua sha*. The shape of the bones where the facial features are located can be uneven, and may prove difficult to scrape. Moreover, beauty is not only on the surface of the skin. It is only by fully stimulating the vitality of the facial skin, veins, flesh, tendons, and bones at all levels that true beautification can be achieved. The deep subcutaneous parts that cause skin problems are diverse, with varying causes and properties. The parts where the scraper penetrates, and the angle and direction of the scraping are also different. Only by mastering the basic techniques of facial *gua sha* and the specific technique for a variety of facial problems can long-term beauty be achieved. The second misunderstanding is only performing facial *gua sha*, and not body conditioning or seeking the root cause. To consolidate the beautifying effect of facial *gua sha*, it is necessary to understand where the spots, acne, and wrinkles on the face indicate where the *qi* (vital energy) and blood are out of balance, and which viscera and organ function has declined. It is only when the *qi* and blood meridians of the corresponding viscera are discriminated and regulated that you can strengthen the beautifying effects of facial *gua sha* on your face.

With a view to spreading the techniques of facial *gua sha* to a wider audience, this book uses accessible language to offer a comprehensive explanation of the techniques for addressing various facial issues. It contains a detailed schematic diagram of *gua sha*, showing the steps to perform it both on yourself and on others. For the first time, the pressure, speed, and angles of *gua sha* are vividly presented in a quantified form through pictures and text. The book also uses theories of traditional Chinese and Western medicine to conduct detailed research and analysis on the key acupoints for facial scraping, and thoroughly explains the key areas of facial beauty and skin care, i.e., the corresponding relationships among the skin structure and acupoints, meridians, *xuan fu* (sweat pores), and holographic acupoint areas where the skin is prone to wrinkles and acne. In this way, readers can identify the symptoms of sub-optimal health in advance from slight changes in facial complexion or small wrinkles. They can then perform facial *gua sha* and comprehensive conditioning of the corresponding viscera and organs, to consolidate the beautifying effect of facial *gua sha*.

Through thousands of cases in clinical practice, it has been proven that if you follow the methods of facial *gua sha* in this book, you will gain unexpected benefits while improving your appearance. Symptoms such as irregular menstruation and dysmenorrhea will be relieved, you will have more energy, and your mood will improve. These gains occur precisely because *gua sha* not only regulates the external skin, but also synchronizes the functions of the internal organs. This is the true meaning of *gua sha* beauty: to work from the outside in, and to beautify from the inside out.

Chapter One
The Principles of Facial *Gua Sha*

In my many years of clinical practice, I often meet a certain type of woman. Their appearance and skin foundation are good, but they have tried many methods to make themselves perfect. Some take medication indiscriminately, which leads to endocrine disorders, and some seek other remedies everywhere after cosmetic methods fail. The truth is, becoming beautiful is very simple. As long as you have an ordinary jade scraper and some simple techniques, you can make your skin glowy. With regular practice and the correct techniques, you can make your facial features more three-dimensional, maintain youth, and delay aging. By scraping the corresponding meridians, acupoints, and holographic acupoints, you will improve your appearance while adjusting the functions of the viscera, making you healthy and beautiful from the inside out.

The skin care products we usually use only stay on the surface of the skin, rarely even penetrating the dermis, let alone reaching the blood and lymphatic systems. *Gua sha* is different. It acts on the dermis of our facial skin, and also penetrates the microcirculation of capillaries (where veins and arteries connect) through the downward pressure of the scraper. At the same time, the focal points of *gua sha* are concentrated on the meridians, acupoints, and holographic acupoints. By scraping these places, we can regulate the functions of the internal organs so as to treat both symptoms and root causes.

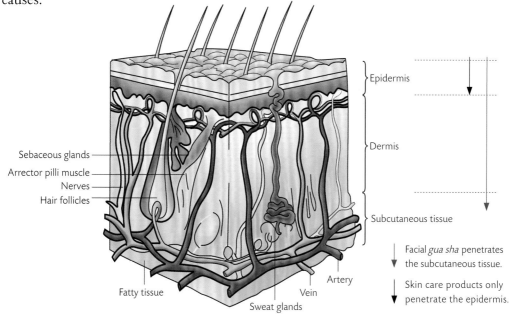

Fig. 1 *Gua sha* can penetrate the microcirculation of the capillaries, solving problems such as a lack of nutrients in the skin, or toxin accumulation.

The Relationship between the Meridians, Viscera, and Facial Beauty

A beautiful face is like a fragrant, lush flower. A beautiful flower must have a sufficient nutrient supply, which relies on the continuous production and delivery of roots and stems. The meridians of the human body are the connectors of the viscera, organs, limbs, and five sense organs. Meridians are like stems that deliver nutrients to flowers, connecting to the viscera on one side and reaching our face on the other, continuously delivering nutrients and conveying information. The viscera are like flower roots, which produce nutrition. If the viscera are unhealthy, it is as if the root of the flower is rotten, being cut off from clean water and rich nourishment. If the meridian is obstructed, it is as if the flower stem is blocked. Flowers lose nutrients and will inevitably wilt and wither, with spots appearing on the leaves and petals. Similarly, with a disorder of *qi* and blood in the meridians and viscera, skin problems can occur such as facial spots, acne, and dullness. This is because the meridians and viscera are closely related to the healthy appearance of the face.

Meridians and Facial Beauty

The *qi* and blood that supply nourishment to our facial skin come from the twelve meridians and the Conception and Governor vessels connected with the five viscera (heart, liver, spleen, lungs, kidneys), and the six *fu*-organs (gallbladder, stomach, small intestine, large intestine, bladder, and *san jiao*—triple energizer). The *qi* of the six *fu*-organs directly connects to the face, while the *qi* of the five viscera ascends to the face through the network vessels connected to the six *fu*-organs. The five viscera are the source of the production and storage of nutrient essence. The six internal organs are the pathways that transport nutrients and metabolic waste, and the meridians are "rivers" full of "boats." Nutrients such as *qi* and blood must be transported through these "rivers" to reach the "plain" of the face, nourishing and cultivating a "pasture." Metabolic waste must also be transported and excreted by the "rivers" to keep the "pasture" clean.

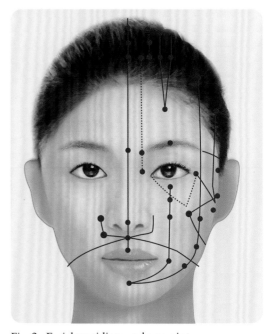

Fig. 2 Facial meridians and acupoints.

The meridians in the body are the pathways through which *qi* and blood run, like road traffic in a city. At intersections, vehicles traveling from south to north gather, leading to accidents that block the normal flow of traffic. If the intersection of meridians and collaterals in the body is congested, stasis of *qi* and blood can occur.

Clean skin is the first element of beauty. Many people suffer from spots, acne, dullness, and large pores on their faces, but the locations where they experience these skin issues vary from person to person. Wrinkles appear on our faces as we age, starting in different places depending on the individual. This is because facial freckles, acne, and wrinkles are all manifestations of dysfunction or weakening of our internal organs. The locations of spots, pimples, and wrinkles are often related to the circulation of meridians. The nature of an individual's bodily cold, heat, deficiency, and excess determines whether they are likely to have facial acne or spots. The difference in the location of meridian dysfunction and the first part to age determine the location of spots, acne, and first wrinkles. If we can understand the law of the relationship between the various problems that appear on the face and the viscera and meridian functions, we can understand our own health status by looking in the mirror every day, and find a cosmetic improvement method to solve the various facial problems with a scraper.

Viscera and Facial Beauty

The relationship between facial skin and viscera is like that between leaves and roots. Nutrition for leaves comes from the roots, while nutrition for the facial skin comes from the viscera, and is regulated and managed by them. The health of the viscera determines the condition of facial skin.

Lungs. The main function of the lungs is to generate and control the basic substance of life activities—*qi*. Through the diffusion of the lungs, the *qi*, blood, and bodily fluids are continuously transported to the skin follicles all over the body, which play the role of nourishing, and regulate the opening of the sweat pores. Whether the skin is moisturized and whether the pores are enlarged is determined by the function of the lungs. If the lungs are dysfunctional and the pores open and close abnormally, the skin will be pale and dull, and the pores will be enlarged due to lack of nourishment and inability to discharge turbid *qi* externally, which will cause acne and other skin conditions.

Spleen, stomach, and intestines. The spleen is the main digestive organ, governing the transportation, transformation, and regulation of the blood. The spleen, stomach, and large and small intestines are responsible for ingesting digested food and absorbing the nutrients in these foods to supply the various tissues and organs of the body. Whether the skin is moist and shiny, and whether the muscles are full and elastic are determined by the function of the spleen. If the spleen, stomach, and large and small intestines are functionally impaired, the muscles and skin will become sallow due to insufficient nutrition; the muscles will be thin, loose, and inelastic, accelerating the aging of the skin and appearance, causing acne and spots, sagging skin, and dry, lackluster hair.

Heart. The main function of the heart is to circulate blood throughout the body, so that nutrients can reach all parts smoothly, ensuring that all tissues and organs have sufficient nutrition and can be free from metabolic waste, keeping the blood clean and healthy. The vitality of the skin is determined by the function of the heart. If the heart function is abnormal, the cells in various parts will suffer problems due to lack of nourishment, making the face dull and dark red, and leading to skin conditions such as chloasma and boils.

Liver. The liver governs the smooth movement of *qi* throughout the body and stores blood. It is an important detoxification organ, and metabolic waste from the internal environment must be sent there for detoxification. Whether the skin is fair, clear, and clean is determined by the function of the liver. When emotions are abnormal or sleep is not good, stagnation of liver *qi* can affect blood circulation and lead to blood stasis. It can also reduce the detoxification ability of the liver, leading to an accumulation of toxins in the blood, which can turn the complexion blue and dark, and lead to pigmentation, acne, allergies, neurodermatitis, gray hair, or hair loss.

Kidneys, bladder. The kidneys govern the growth and development of the entire body, including the skin. The kidneys store and provide the innate essence most needed for the growth and development of various parts of the human body. Together with the bladder, they complete water metabolism, metabolize beneficial bodily fluids, filter harmful substances in bodily fluids, and produce and discharge wastewater (urine). The innate genetic factors in the kidney determine a person's basic skin quality, skin color, and aging speed. The strength of the kidney function will directly affect whether the hair is full-colored, whether the hearing is sensitive, and the aging degree of facial bones and skin. Excessive metabolites in the body caused by kidney *qi* deficiency can cause a dull complexion, brown spots, age spots, and edema. In individuals with osteoporosis due to kidney deficiency, the facial bones atrophy prematurely, the aging of the skin is accelerated, and wrinkles are formed early.

The face is also a monitor of the health of our internal organs. The sages of traditional Chinese medicine discovered through practice that there is a one-to-one correspondence between the face and viscera. Modern biological holographic theory also confirms that each local organ of the human body with relatively independent boundaries, and relatively independent structure and function, is the epitome of the whole. Therefore, the face is the holographic miniature of the human body. Observing it can allow us to understand the health of the internal organs.

The holographic distribution of the face is regular. The head, face, neck, and torso are in the middle, and the limbs are distributed on both sides. The distribution of various organs in the body is like a human figure with outstretched arms and legs, which is completely consistent with the records in the *Inner Canon of the Yellow Emperor* (*Huangdi Neijing*)—a classical Chinese medical text. According to the theory of biological holography, the parts of the face corresponding to various viscera and organs have a holographic corresponding relationship with the specific viscera and organs, where the well-being or ailments of each facial region mirror the health or diseases of their corresponding internal organs. In traditional Chinese medicine, the meridians connect the viscera internally, connect the skin externally, and connect upward to the face, which provides a new theoretical basis for holographic correspondence from another perspective.

Whether from the records of the *Inner Canon of the Yellow Emperor* or from modern biological holographic theory, it can be concluded that the upper, middle, and lower parts of the face correspond to the head, face, heart and lungs, liver, gallbladder, spleen

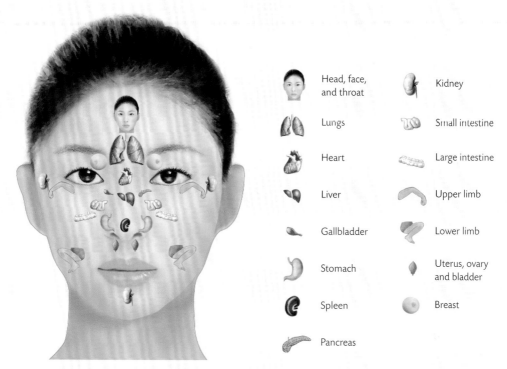

	Head, face, and throat		Kidney
	Lungs		Small intestine
	Heart		Large intestine
	Liver		Upper limb
	Gallbladder		Lower limb
	Stomach		Uterus, ovary and bladder
	Spleen		Breast
	Pancreas		

Fig. 3   Facial holographic acupoint areas.

and stomach, genitourinary organs, with the viscera positioned in the middle, and limbs on the outside. The color, luster, and shape of the three parts can be compared to analyze the differences. Judging by the part of the face that has the most severe problem, the most severely damaged part of the body can be identified through holographic comparison.

What Is Cosmetic Holographic Meridian *Gua Sha*?

The reason why facial *gua sha* is applied on the skin but can regulate the skin, meridians, and internal organs at the same time is due to the support of meridian theory and biological holographic theory. The meridians are the basis for the diagnosis and treatment of various therapies in traditional Chinese medicine. According to TCM, meridians are the pathways that carry the whole body's *qi* and blood, network the internal organs, limbs, and joints, and communicate with the body's internal and external environment.

   The method of selecting the scraping area according to the main rule of meridians and acupoints is called the "meridian scraping method." Facial *gua sha* uses the theory of meridians to diagnose and analyze facial problems, and then scrape the face and body according to the pathways of meridians and principles of acupoint treatment.

   "Holographic" means "containing all information." The bio-holographic theory points out that the part contains all the information of the whole. The technique of using bio-holographic theory to guide *gua sha* scraping, and to select specific organs for *gua sha* scraping treatment, diagnosis, and cosmetic improvement is called the "holographic scraping method."

When the two are combined, they are referred to as the "holographic meridian scraping method for cosmetic improvement and wellness." This is a cosmetic TCM technique targeting the beauty-damaging skin conditions that appear on the human face, using special scraping tools and media, along with a variety of scraping techniques for the face and body, and performing dialectical scraping and conditioning.

Holographic meridian scraping method starts from the skin, meridians, and viscera. It cleans the blood, unblocks the meridians, and promotes skin metabolism to achieve beauty. This kind of beauty is different from superficial make-up. Make-up is just a cover-up. Scraping for cosmetic improvement regulates *qi* and blood, improves microcirculation, cleans the internal environment, and can remove endotoxins and other metabolic waste deposited in the deep layer of the skin, dredging the nutrients-supplying channels to skin cells. This improves the *qi* and blood supply of the face, activates and restores the physiological functions of the facial skin itself, and at the same time stimulates the body's regulating function to achieve the optimal state, delay aging, and restore natural beauty.

Holographic meridian scraping method alleviates both symptoms and root causes by simultaneously regulating the viscera, the *qi* and blood, and the face, achieving both beauty and health. Because of its simplicity of use, remarkable results, and lack of side effects, it is called the quintessence of cosmetic TCM techniques.

Why does the scraping tools have such a great stimulating effect? The *xuan fu* mentioned in the classical works of TCM may have the answer.

Xuan fu is a term used in TCM to describe human tissues, first seen in the *Inner Canon of the Yellow Emperor*. In recent years, some scholars have come to believe that it has both broad and narrow meanings. The narrow sense refers to the so-called sweat pores, and the broad sense refers to tiny pores and their channel structures all over the human body. *Xuan fu* is the site where the tissue cells of the body carry out metabolism and obtain nutrition, and it is also the site for function regulation, bodily fluid, information transmission, and conversion.

Modern research has identified that there are a large number of microcirculation, lymph, and peripheral nerves in the circulation site of the meridians. The location and function of *xuan fu* are very similar to microcirculation and peripheral nerves in modern medicine. The pressing force of scraping stimulates the *xuan fu* of the affected parts, thereby promoting microcirculation and lymphatic circulation, and smoothing the movement of *qi*.

Key Areas of Facial *Gua Sha*

In TCM, the skin of the face is divided into regions, each managed by one of the meridians running in this region. Each meridian manages the part where it is located and the parts to the surrounding meridian area, like a series of rivers, irrigating and nourishing lives in different basins. The management scope of each meridian is called the cutaneous region of this meridian in TCM, and the command center that it manages is made up of the acupoints. They are responsible for delivering nutrients to the skin and surrounding tissues and organs, carrying away waste, responding freely to the various stimuli of the internal and external environment on the skin and surrounding tissues and organs and ensuring the safety of the body's internal environment and external barriers. The meridians, cutaneous regions, and acupoints fulfill their duties, nurturing the beauty of the face.

The acupoints are very sensitive to changes in the internal environment and visceral organs, and can reflect these changes on the surface of the skin, in the form of skin conditions and problems. In this way, the facial skin is a monitor of the internal environment. At the same time, acupoints have important feedback and regulation functions. Scraping and stimulating the cutaneous regions and acupoints can incite their functions, transmit positive information, drive away pathogenic factors, repair and maintain the normal physiological functions of the skin and various tissues and organs, and keep them in the best condition.

Facial Acupoints

The acupoints are the special parts of the body where the *qi* of the internal organs and meridians is infused in and out. They are both reaction points to diseases and stimulation points for acupuncture, moxibustion, pressing, and scraping. The effect of facial *gua sha* is very good, because the acupuncture points commonly used have the function of infusing *qi* and blood and reflecting pathological conditions. They are also the starting and ending points of our facial muscles, as well as key points of blood and lymph circulation and nerve regulation.

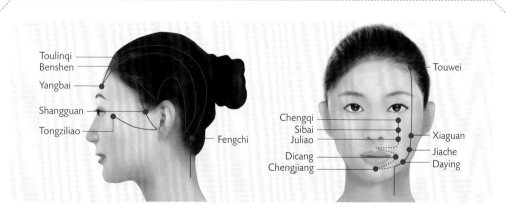

Fig. 4   The commonly used acupoints for facial *gua sha* have TCM health benefits. They are also the starting and ending points of the facial muscles and fascia, and the regulatory points for blood, lymph, and nerves. Stimulating these points can promote the recovery of muscle elasticity, remove excess bodily fluid, and accelerate the skin's metabolism.

Scraping, pressing and kneading these key acupoints promotes lymphatic circulation and blood circulation. It also enhances the elasticity of muscles, increases the flexibility of the fascia, and adjusts the sensitivity of the nerves. Through these subtle adjustments, the facial muscles are fully stretched and contracted, the elasticity of stretching is enhanced, and the slackness of the skin is changed, thereby changing the perception of our external appearance.

Facial Muscles

Understanding the distribution, shape, and function of the muscles is of great help in achieving good effects using facial *gua sha* for cosmetic improvement, face thinning, and wrinkle removal.

The facial skin is thin, soft, and elastic, and contains a high concentration of sebaceous glands, sweat glands, and hair follicles. There is more fat in the cheeks, and the subcutaneous fat in the eyelids is less and loose. If there is edema, it will appear in these parts first.

The facial muscles are skin muscles, which are thin and slender. They start from the bones or fascia of the face and cranium, and end at the skin. When these muscles contract, they directly affect the skin and produce facial expressions. The facial muscles are mostly located around the eyes, lips, and nostrils. According to the arrangement and function of the muscle fibers, they are usually divided into two types: circular muscles and radial muscles. The former plays a role in closure. The latter plays a role in

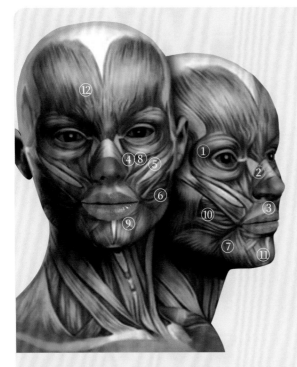

① Orbicularis oculi——crow's feet

② Nasalis muscle——frown lines, wrinkles in the middle of the nose bridge

③ Orbicularis oris——upper lip lines, nasolabial folds

④ Levator labii superioris

⑤ Musculi zygomaticus

⑥ Risorius

⑦ Depressor anguli oris

⑧ Levator anguli oris——eye bag lines

⑨ Depressor labii inferioris——lower lip lines

⑩ Buccal muscles——nasolabial folds

⑪ Mentalis——lower lip lines

⑫ Frontalis muscles——wrinkles on the forehead

Expression lines, ——nasolabial folds, eye bag lines

Fig. 5 Facial muscles and associated wrinkles.

expanding. The facial muscles are innervated by the facial nerve. The acupoints in the meridians of TCM, especially the facial acupoints, are mostly located at the start and end points of facial muscles and fascia, and the circulation of many meridians is also consistent with the direction of the muscle fibers. The muscle fibers of the facial muscles and the elastic fibers in the superficial fascia are connected with the corium layer to form the natural creases or wrinkles of the skin. When the facial muscles relax, corresponding wrinkles will appear on the face. The acupoints are like the tightness switches on the start and end points of the muscles. Stimulating these points causes the muscles to tighten and contract.

Facial Meridians

The meridians that pass through the face are the Governor Vessel, Conception Vessel, Taiyang Bladder Meridian of Foot (BL), Shaoyang Gallbladder Meridian of Foot (GB), Shaoyang Triple Energizer Meridian of Hand (TE), Yangming Large Intestine Meridian of Hand (LI), Yangming Stomach Meridian of Foot (ST), Taiyang Small Intestine Meridian of Hand (SI), and Jueyin Liver Meridian of Foot (LR). Scraping these meridians and their main acupoints can have therapeutic and cosmetic effects.

Governor Vessel. Facial circulation area: Goes down along the forehead to the nasal column and the philtrum, down to the lower jaw, surrounds the lips, and connects to the center under the eyes.

Main acupoints: ① Suliao acupoint: In the center of the nose tip. ② Duiduan acupoint: At the midpoint of the upper lip. ③ Renzhong acupoint: At the intersection of the upper third and middle third of the philtrum.

Areas of responsibility and the effects of facial *gua sha*: In charge of the midline of forehead, middle of the nose, and philtrum. Scraping the Governor Vessel can activate lip muscle tissue, improve wrinkles, moisturize skin and lips, and lighten dark spots.

Conception Vessel. Facial circulation area: Goes up through the throat to the inside of the lower lip, surrounds the lips, goes up to the Yinjiao acupoint, meets the Governor Vessel, and branches up to the eyes.

Main acupoints: ① Chengjiang acupoint: First find the mentolabial sulcus on the chin (the shallow groove under the

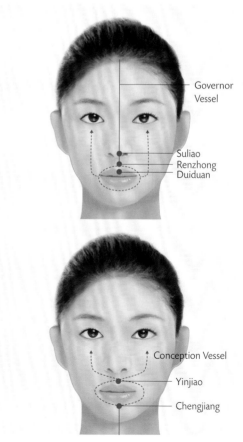

Governor Vessel

Suliao
Renzhong
Duiduan

Conception Vessel

Yinjiao

Chengjiang

lower lip and in the center of the chin). The acupoint is in the central depression of the mentolabial sulcus.

Areas of responsibility and the effects of facial *gua sha*: In charge of the areas going around the lips and branches up to the eyes. The orbicularis oris is under the Conception Vessel. Scraping the Conception Vessel on the face can stimulate the contraction of the orbicularis oris, eliminate the dullness of the lower lip and lower jaw, dilute pigmentation, and reduce lower lip lines and nasolabial folds.

Taiyang Bladder Meridian of Foot. Facial circulation area: From the Jingming acupoints on the inner canthus of the eyes to the middle of the forehead.

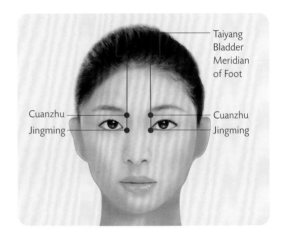

Main acupoints: ① Jingming acupoint: Slightly above the inner corner of the eyes and close to the eyeball. ② Cuanzhu acupoint: In the depression at the inner end of the eyebrows.

Areas of responsibility and the effects of facial *gua sha*: In charge of the inner corner of the eyes, and the forehead. Under the Taiyang Bladder Meridian of Foot are the adducens oculi muscle, frontalis muscles, and corrugator supercilii. Scraping the Taiyang Bladder Meridian of Foot on the face will help stimulate the contraction of these muscles and improve frown lines, wrinkles in the middle of the nose bridge, dark circles, dullness on the forehead, chloasma, dry eyes, and eye fatigue.

Shaoyang Gallbladder Meridian of Foot. Facial circulation area: From the outer corner of the eye to the front of the ear, up to the frontal angle, from the lateral head to both sides of the forehead.

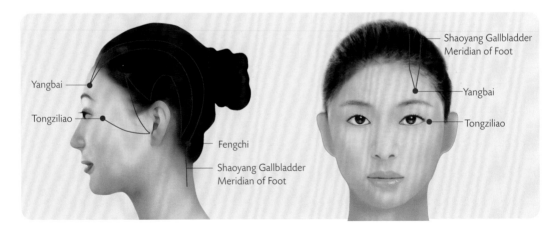

Main acupoints: ① Yangbai acupoint: In the forehead, looking straight ahead with your eyes level, straight up from the pupils, one cun above the eyebrows. ② Tongziliao acupoint: First, find the outer corner of the eye, and touch outward across the orbit. Its lateral edge is the Tongziliao acupoint. ③ Fengchi acupoint: Under the occipital bone, in the depression between the sternocleidomastoid muscle and the upper end of the trapezius muscle.

Areas of responsibility and the effects of facial *gua sha*: In charge of the outer corners of the eyes, the forehead angles, areas around both ears and both sides of the forehead. Under the Shaoyang Gallbladder Meridian of Foot are the ends of the orbicularis oculi, frontalis muscles, and buccal muscles. Stimulating the Gallbladder Meridian can activate, brighten, and moisten the skin in the Gallbladder Meridian area, lift the corners of the eyes, reduce wrinkles, and lighten pigmentation.

Shaoyang Triple Energizer Meridian of Hand. Facial circulation area: In front of the ears, through the Shangguan acupoint (see location in the Appendix) to the outer corner of the eyes.

Main acupoints: ① Sizhukong acupoint: At the outer edge of the eyebrows, in the depression at the tip of the eyebrows.

Areas of responsibility and the effects of facial *gua sha*: In charge of the front of the ear to the outer corner of the eye, and the orbicularis oculi. Scraping this area can brighten, moisten, and lift the skin of the eyebrows and outer parts, reduce wrinkles, and lighten dark spots.

Yangming Large Intestine Meridian of Hand. Facial circulation area: Goes up from the neck through the cheeks, into the lower gums, back around to the upper lip, then crisscrosses over the philtrum, and is distributed on both sides of the nostrils.

Main acupoints: ① Yingxiang acupoint: On the outer edge of the wings of nose, in the nasolabial fold. ② Kouheliao acupoint: On the upper lip, directly below the outer edge of the nostrils, parallel to the upper third of the nasolabial fold.

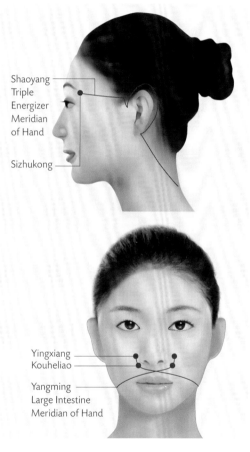

Areas of responsibility and the effects of facial *gua sha*: In charge of area above the upper lip, both sides of the nose wings, and the philtrum; the starting point of the orbicularis oris and the buccinator muscle. Scraping can refine the skin, shrink pores, slow down the development of nasolabial folds, and improve the corners of the mouth.

Yangming Stomach Meridian of Foot. Facial circulation area: Starts from the Chengqi acupoint under the eyes and goes down along the outer side of the nasal column, enters the upper teeth and then goes out, surrounds the lips, intersects at the lip groove, retreats and goes down along the lower jaw bone. It then goes up along the mandibular angle and passes through the front of the ears, going along the hairline to the front of the forehead.

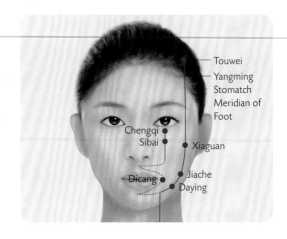

Main acupoints: ① Chengqi acupoint: Vertically downward from the midpoint of the pupil, the point where it intersects with the horizontal line at the lower edge of the eye socket is the Chengqi acupoint. ② Sibai acupoint: Vertically downward from the Chengqi acupoint, the Sibai acupoint is the depression on the cheekbones. ③ Dicang acupoint: Vertically downward from the midpoint of the pupil, the point where it intersects with the horizontal line at the corner of the mouth is the Dicang acupoint. ④ Daying acupoint: With teeth clenched, feel from the corner of the mouth to the lower front edge of the tense muscles, the place where the facial artery pulses is the Daying acupoint. ⑤ Jiache acupoint: With teeth clenched, there is a tense and raised muscle at the highest point on the cheek, press it and then relax—this is the Jiache point. ⑥ Xiaguan acupoint: On the face, in the depression between the center of the lower edge of the zygomatic arch and the mandibular notch. ⑦ Touwei acupoint: Take the horizontal line 0.5 cun above the hairline of the frontal angle as the x-axis, and the vertical line 4.5 cun away from the midline of the head as the y-axis, the place where the two axes intersect is the Touwei acupoint.

Areas of responsibility and the effects of facial *gua sha*: In charge of the center of the lower eyelid downward, the lips, the lateral sides of the cheek, the lateral sides of the forehead, and the bottom of the cheek, covering almost all the facial muscles. Scraping the acupoints of the Stomach Meridian can reduce bags under the eyes, soften the nasolabial folds, tighten the skin, refine pores, lift and thin the face, moisten the lips, and improve a dark yellow complexion.

Taiyang Small Intestine Meridian of Hand. Facial circulation area: From both sides of the front of the neck to the cheek area, the inner and outer corners of the eyes, and to the front of the ears.

Main acupoints: ① Quanliao acupoint: In the depression on the lower edge of the cheekbone directly below the outer corner of the eye. ② Tinggong acupoint: In the depression in front of the tragus when the mouth is open.

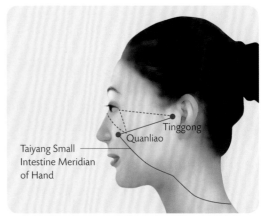

Areas of responsibility and the effects of facial *gua sha*: In charge of the cheekbones, the inner and outer corners of the eyes, the buccal muscle, and the orbicularis oculi. Scraping the Quanliao acupoint can make the complexion rosy, improve redness, lighten pigmentation, tighten the skin, slim and lift the face, and prevent cheek acne.

Jueyin Liver Meridian of Foot.
Facial circulation area: From the eye sockets to the forehead, down to the cheeks, and around the lips.

Main acupoints: ① Midpoint of the upper and lower eye sockets: Under the Yuyao acupoint, in the depression of the upper orbital bone, under the Chengqi acupoint, in the depression of the lower orbital bone.

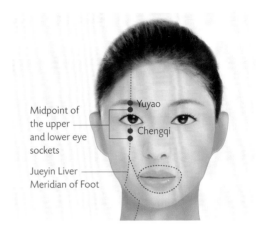

Areas of responsibility and the effects of facial *gua sha*: In charge of the eye system, both sides of the forehead, the cheeks, the orbicularis oris, the frontalis muscles, and the buccal muscles. Scraping the Liver Meridian area can improve the skin color on both sides of the forehead and cheeks, lighten spots, reduce wrinkles and eye bags, and improve dark circles, dry eyes, and eye fatigue.

Organs Corresponding to the Facial Areas

Head and face area. On the upper half of the forehead, corresponding to the brain, reflecting psychological pressure and the state of the *qi* and blood in the heart and brain.

Facial problems and their significance: Deficiency-cold people (with vital *qi* deficiency and internal cold) are often lacking in luster in this area; excessive use of the brain produces premature horizontal wrinkles in this area.

Lung and throat area. The area from the middle of the lower half of the forehead to the top of the eyebrows is the lung and throat area, and the corresponding organs are the throat and lungs, reflecting the function of the respiratory system and the abundance and deficiency of *qi*.

Facial problems and their significance: Small, light-colored acne indicates the flaring up of deficient fire of the lungs, often accompanied by chronic pharyngitis; redness of the skin in the lung area can indicate high blood pressure in the middle-aged and above; dark color and less luster is a deficiency of lung *qi*, and a lower concavity means a longer-term deficiency of lung *qi*.

Heart area. The area between the eyes is the heart area, which corresponds to the heart and reflects its health.

Facial problems and their significance: Premature horizontal wrinkles between the eyebrows indicate insufficient heart *qi* and blood; a lack of luster indicates heart *qi* deficiency, and dull or blue skin color indicates a stagnation of heart blood.

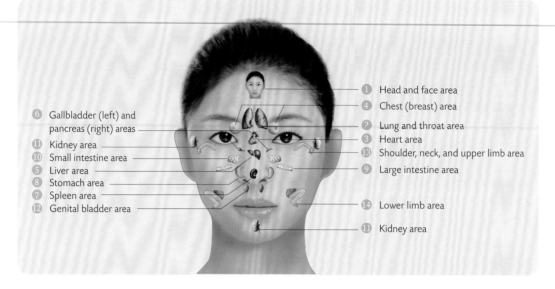

6 Gallbladder (left) and
 pancreas (right) areas
11 Kidney area
10 Small intestine area
5 Liver area
8 Stomach area
7 Spleen area
12 Genital bladder area

1 Head and face area
4 Chest (breast) area
2 Lung and throat area
3 Heart area
13 Shoulder, neck, and upper limb area
9 Large intestine area

14 Lower limb area

11 Kidney area

Chest (breast) area. The area from both sides of the nose root to the inner lower part of the eyebrows.

Facial problems and their significance: People with a full and bulging shape in this area should be alert to breast hyperplasia and breast disorders.

Liver area. The middle of the nose bridge, corresponding to the liver and reflecting its health.

Facial problems and their significance: A lack of luster in the middle of the nose indicates liver *qi* deficiency; longitudinal fine lines indicate liver and kidney deficiency which means you need to strengthen lumbar spine health care; a dull color indicates liver depression and *qi* stagnation, there's a risk of fatty liver.

Gallbladder and pancreas areas. The left side of the middle of the nose bridge is the pancreas area, and the right side is the gallbladder area, reflecting the health of the two organs respectively.

Facial problems and their significance: A lack of luster or a dark blue tinge in the middle part of the nose and the right gallbladder area suggests a deficiency of liver and gallbladder *qi*, liver depression and *qi* stagnation. If the left side of the middle of the nose is obviously lacking luster, or is dark or stained, this indicates that pancreatic function is reduced.

Spleen and stomach areas. The tip of the nose and both sides of the nose respectively reflect the health of the spleen and stomach.

Facial problems and their significance: A lack of luster on the tip of the nose indicates spleen *qi* deficiency; large pores and a lack of luster on the tip of the nose indicate spleen deficiency over time; a dull blue nose indicates cold pain in the abdomen; an oily nose, redness, or rosacea indicates dampness-heat of the spleen and stomach; a red nosewing and nasal fossa or acne indicates stomach heat, dark red indicates stagnated stomach heat with blood stasis; pale nosewing with a lack of luster indicate stomach *qi* deficiency and stomach cold.

Large intestine area. The area from the pupil and the lower side of the outer corner of the eyes to the lower side of the cheekbones next to the nose, reflecting the health of the large intestine.

Facial problems and their significance: A lack of luster or large pores in this area indicate large intestine *qi* deficiency; acne indicates large intestine heat exuberance; chloasma indicates large intestine *qi* stagnation and long-term blood stasis.

Small intestine area. The area under the inner corner of the eyes and the pupils, above the inner and upper part of the cheekbones, reflecting the health of the small intestine.

Facial problems and their significance: A lack of luster or large pores in this area indicate small intestine *qi* deficiency; acne indicates small intestine heat exuberance; chloasma indicates long-term small intestines *qi* stagnation and blood stasis; redness indicates a deficiency of heart *qi* and blood stasis.

Kidney and genital bladder areas. Both sides above the upper lip correspond to the bladder area; the middle of the philtrum, corresponds to the uterus area for women, the prostate area for men, and both sides of the upper lip correspond to the ovaries for women, reflecting the health of the reproductive organs. The Chengjiang acupoint at the lower part of the lower lip corresponds to the kidneys and also reflects the health of the uterus. Another corresponding part of the kidney area is the lateral cheek area in front of the ears.

Facial problems and their significance: A red upper lip or acne, accompanied by yellow urine, indicate bladder heat; dull blue skin around the upper and lower lips indicate kidney *yang* deficiency, and deficiency-cold in the lower *jiao*; constant acne below the lower lip and on the jaw indicates heat and dampness in the lower *jiao*, suggesting endocrine disorders and ovarian conditions in women; horizontal wrinkles on the lower jaw indicate kidney deficiency and lower back pain; dull color, a lack of luster and chloasma on the cheek area in front of the ears indicate kidney deficiency.

Shoulder, neck, and upper limb area. Below the outer corner of the eyes, above the cheekbones.

Facial problems and their significance: A lack of luster under the outer corners of the eyes, or premature sagging, or longitudinal wrinkles indicate insufficient *qi* and blood in the neck and shoulders, weakened muscle strength in the neck and shoulders, and even soreness in the neck and shoulders; the appearance of chloasma in the upper limb area is a result of *qi* stagnation and blood stasis in the neck and shoulder area, and neck and shoulder pain.

Lower limb area. On the outside of the lips, below the cheekbones.

Facial problems and their significance: A lack of luster, premature sagging, or longitudinal wrinkles in the lower limb area indicates that the lower limbs have insufficient *qi* and blood, weakened muscle strength, and knee joint pain; the appearance of chloasma in the lower limb area is due to deficiency-cold in the lower limbs, *qi* stagnation and blood stasis, and pain in the knee joint.

Self-Diagnosing Skin Abnormalities

The key to facial *gua sha* is to use the scraper to identify the reason for unsightly skin problems and find the crux of the issue. By looking for abnormal changes under the skin, i.e., positive reactions, and communicating with the body, we can perceive the earliest distress signals from the meridians and viscera, and then use scrapers to respond.

Discovering Positive Reactions

One of the main characteristics and advantages of scraping is that it can quickly find the key points that affect beauty, that is, the early distress signals sent by the meridians and acupoints. The scraper is used to apply a certain pressure to scrape the skin. Under normal circumstances, the scraping is smooth and there should be no pain on the skin. An astringent feeling to the skin, subcutaneous grit-like nodular tissue, muscle tension, stiffness, relaxation, atrophy, an abnormal temperature, and pain are all positive reactions.

These positive reactions are precisely the manifestations of poor circulation of the meridians, acupoints, and *xuan fu*, which can exist on the face or various parts of the body, impeding the flow of *qi* and blood and affecting the function of the internal organs, leading to subhealth and facial aesthetic disorders. If we understand the relationship between the various positive reactions and health and beauty, and learn the rules, we will be able to identify the causes of unsightly facial problems, and tips for facial *gua sha*.

Diagnostic Rules for Positive Reactions

The key to facial *gua sha* is to find the following positive reaction points, and use scraping techniques to gradually reduce and eliminate these positive reactions. In doing so, *qi* and blood in the meridians will flow smoothly, the viscera will function normally, and the face will have sufficient *qi* and blood, leading to natural cosmetic improvement.

Haptic Perception	Specific Results	Indications
Temperature change	Warm and cozy	*Qi* and blood in the meridians or tissue and organs are unobstructed.
	Cold	Meridians or tissue and organs feel cold pathogen.
Skin tactility	Moisturized and elastic	*Qi* and blood in the meridians or tissue and organs are unobstructed, and nutrition is sufficient.
	Dry, astringent	Meridians or tissue and organs have ischemia, hypoxia, and mostly *yin* deficiency, bodily fluid deficiency.
	Nail-file feeling	Blood stasis syndrome from *qi* and blood stasis in meridians or tissue and organs over time and there's a lack of nutrition.

Haptic Perception	Specific Results	Indications
Skin tactility	Greasy feeling	*Qi* and blood in the meridians or tissue and organs have phlegm-dampness syndrome or dampness-heat syndrome, which is caused by phlegm-dampness or damp-heat blocking collaterals.
Pain	Soreness	*Qi* and blood deficiency in the meridians or tissue and organs.
	Swelling pain	*Qi* stagnation in meridians or tissue and organs, *qi* movement is obstructed.
	Stabbing pain	Blood stasis in the meridians or tissue and organs.
Grit-like tissue under the skin	Only grit-like tissue	Meridians or tissue and organs form lesions due to *qi* stagnation and blood stasis, or previous lesions have no symptoms at present.
	Coexistence of grit-like tissue and pain	Slight inflammatory changes in meridians or tissue and organs, or symptoms due to a disorder of *qi* and blood in the meridians.
Subcutaneous nodular tissue	Nodular tissue only	A previous inflammatory reaction locally, but the symptoms have disappeared.
	Coexistence of nodular tissue and pain	The meridians or tissue and organs have had *qi* and blood stasis for a long time, or there are local inflammatory changes, with current symptoms.
Muscle tension	Tense, stiff	Ischemia and hypoxia in the meridians or tissue and organs; mostly excess syndrome (symptoms manifested due to an excess of pathogenic energy).
	Slack, atrophy	Ischemia and hypoxia in meridians or tissue and organs; mostly deficiency syndrome (syndrome of weakness caused by insufficient essence, nutrients and blood, or deficiency syndrome of viscera).

Facial skin texture, color, and features are determined by innate genetic factors. What facial *gua sha* aims to achieve is to restore the pure and natural beauty of facial skin, bring it to its best condition, delay the speed of aging of the skin and facial features, and solve common problems. So what beautifying effects can scraping achieve?

One is to nourish and rejuvenate the skin, and delay aging. Frequent facial *gua sha* can regulate the secretions of the sebaceous glands and sweat glands, enhance the self-cleaning function of the pores, clean the skin, promote skin metabolism, cleansing the skin, refining the pores, moisturizing the skin and delaying the skin-aging process.

The second is to brighten the skin and remove freckles. Facial *gua sha* can promote blood circulation to the facial skin, open the *xuan fu*, remove metabolites in the blood, improve dull skin color, dilute chloasma and freckles, and revitalize the skin's original clear and clean natural color.

The third is to improve skin problems, and eliminate spots and wrinkles. Scraping the key acupoints on the face can improve dark circles and redness, prevent and reduce eyebags, relieve or prevent wrinkles, and reduce acne marks.

The fourth is to slim the face, and enhance and tighten the skin. The correct facial *gua sha* method can improve the circulation of blood and lymph, drain excess water, and have an obvious slimming effect on a swollen face. It can also enhance the elasticity of facial muscles and the flexibility of fascia to achieve firmness, lifting the facial skin, preventing and improving drooping corners of the eyes and mouth.

The fifth is to remove acne and promote facial health. The combination of facial *gua sha* and body *gua sha* can consolidate the immediate beautifying effect of facial *gua sha*. Body *gua sha* can also provide a fundamental solution, treating facial acne.

The Four Elements of *Gua Sha*

If you want to use facial *gua sha* to improve the appearance of your face without producing *sha* (red and purplish-red freckles and spots on the skin), you must master certain techniques. Correct facial *gua sha* should be a comfortable and enjoyable process as well as a way of achieving beautifying results. To this end, you need to master the four elements of *gua sha*, namely speed, intensity, angle, and time.

Speed

Speed refers to the rhythm of scraping. Slow scraping speed is a major feature of facial *gua sha*, and fast scraping is highly discouraged. Slowness is the key to avoiding producing *sha*, fading and removing freckles, and increasing comfort. The correct scraping speed should be controlled. It is advisable to scrape 2 to 3 times within one calm breath.

Intensity

Intensity refers to the pressing force into the skin when scraping. For facial *gua sha*, the scraping consists of a pressing force deep into the skin—never rubbing only on the surface, as surface friction has no cosmetic effect and also damages the skin, resulting in epidermal edema. The correct technique is to make contact with the skin using the scraper, and use pressing force to gently penetrate down to the subcutaneous tissue or deep into the muscle, instead of pressing down forcefully. The pressure differs depending on the purpose of the scraping: For facial skincare and soothing fine wrinkles, the pressure should be enough to reach the subcutaneous soft tissue layer below the epidermis and above the muscles; for diagnosis, finding and eliminating positive reactions, and slimming the face, the pressure should reach the deeper muscles within the epidermis and above the bones.

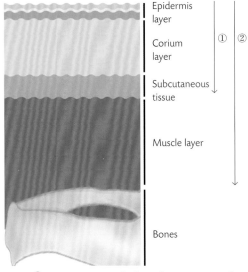

Fig. 6 ① Pressure to reach the subcutaneous soft tissue layer. ② Pressure to reach the deep muscle layer above the bones.

Angle

This refers to the angle formed between the plane of the scraper and the skin when scraping. Generally, the smaller the angle, the more comfortable it is to scrape. For facial scraping, use the edge or the plane of the scraper to touch the skin. The angle between the

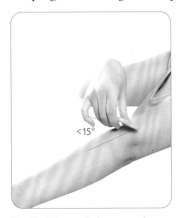

Fig. 7 The angle between the scraper and the skin is less than 15 degrees.

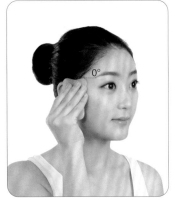

Fig. 8 The angle between the scraper and the skin is zero degree.

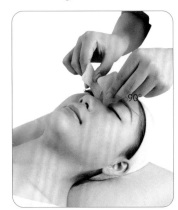

Fig. 9 Vertical-pressing and kneading on the Jingming acupoint should be kept at 90 degrees.

plane of the scraper and the skin should be less than 15 degrees. When the plane touches the skin, the angle could even be zero degrees (except for the Jingming acupoint of the eyes).

Time

This refers to the length of time for scraping, which is divided into local scraping time for each part and overall scraping time. Generally, each part is gently scraped 15 to 20 times. Timing should be reduced appropriately for sensitive skin.

There are two methods of facial scraping: skin care, and diagnosis and treatment.

To maintain the facial skin or when scraping frequently, go from the forehead to the jaw. Scrape each part 3 to 5 times each time, 2 to 3 times within one calm breath, for a total of 10 to 15 minutes.

When scraping the face for diagnosis, each part needs to be scraped 5 to 10 times each time in order. Facial scraping for slimming only works on key parts with special lifting techniques, 2 to 3 strokes at a normal breathing speed, for 10 to 20 minutes each time. For whitening and anti-freckle treatment or when the scraping interval is long, each part needs to be scraped 5 to 10 times each time in order, for no longer than 30 to 40 minutes. A comprehensive scraping session can be performed once a week. When scraping a single area, such as around the eyes, forehead, or around the mouth for targeted treatment such as freckle removal and wrinkle reduction, scrape the specific part 10 to 15 times each time, once a day.

For people with a rosy complexion or thin, oily, or sensitive skin, loose muscles, and poor elasticity, and for the elderly, the pressure of scraping should be reduced appropriately. Each part should be scraped 3 to 4 times each time, and the overall scraping time should be shortened as appropriate. For thicker skin, skin with good elasticity, young people, and those with sallow or dull skin, the pressure should be increased appropriately, and each part should be scraped 5 times each time. The overall scraping time should be extended as well, but no more than 50 minutes.

Precautions

When performing facial *gua sha*, the following precautions should be observed:

1. Avoid wind when scraping. The room temperature must be above 18°C. Avoid cold air and direct air conditioning.

2. When scraping in the lying position, cover the body parts with cotton and wool fabrics according to the room temperature, and keep warm.

3. When cleaning the facial skin before scraping, it is strictly forbidden to use facial cleansers containing exfoliating or softening agents that work on the keratin layers. Facial *gua sha* must be preceded by applying facial *gua sha* cream. Direct scraping of the skin without applying lubricant is strictly prohibited.

4. Scrape in the direction of the muscle fibers, and pay attention to maintaining an upward lifting direction and strength at all times.

5. Areas of facial acne and folliculitis should not be scraped.

6. People who have completed an exfoliation treatment should not undergo facial scraping for 28 days.

7. During pregnancy, the Renzhong and Chengjiang acupoints must not be scraped.

8. Use discretion to scrape lightly or avoid scraping areas with red blood streaks.

9. After scraping the face, if you need to apply a mask, wash your face with warm water, and warm the mask before applying it. If you need to go out, avoid outdoor activities until half an hour after facial scraping.

10. After a scraping treatment, drink a cup of hot water to rehydrate and encourage the discharge of metabolites.

In addition, since *gua sha* therapy is used to treat skin conditions and beautify the skin, pressure must be applied deep into the skin, which has a certain compression effect on blood vessels. The *sha* produced by scraping must be metabolized by the immune cells, liver, and kidneys, so facial *gua sha* is not suitable for:

1. People with severe cardiovascular and cerebrovascular conditions, poor liver and kidney function, or other serious conditions.

2. People with illnesses with a tendency to bleed, such as thrombocytopenia, leukemia, and allergic purpura.

3. Menstruating women, to avoid aggravating bleeding. During pregnancy, the lower abdomen, Renzhong, Chengjiang and other acupoints that may cause a miscarriage must not be scraped.

4. People with anemia.

5. Those who have suffered a fracture or acute soft tissue injury. The injured part of the tendon and ligament must not be scraped.

Preparation

The preparations for facial *gua sha* include the choice of environment, comfortable beds, chairs, special scraping tools, and facial cleansing supplies. Facial *gua sha* is generally better in an indoor environment, either sitting or lying. When performing facial *gua sha* for others, it is best to scrape in the lying position in an environment with a suitable temperature. It is advisable to control the indoor temperature at 18 to 26°C for body scraping. When the room temperature is too high, avoid direct blowing of air-conditioning or fan air. When the room temperature is low, cover up with clothes, blankets, or towels to keep warm.

Special Facial *Gua Sha* Tools

There are five tools needed for facial *gua sha*: jade facial *gua sha* scraper, jade facial *gua sha* scraper for eyes, jade *gua sha* scraper for body, scraping comb, and holographic scraper. There is also facial *gua sha* cream and scraping oil for skin protection and lubrication.

Scrapers for facial *gua sha* and for body are mostly made of jade. According to the *Compendium of Materia Medica*, jade has a sweet taste and neutral nature, enters the Taiyin Lung Meridian of Hand, moistens the heart and lungs, and clears lung heat. Jade contains a variety of trace elements needed by the human body, and has the functions of nourishing *yin* and clearing heat, nourishing and calming the mind, promoting fitness and curing illnesses. Jade has a moisturizing and nourishing effect on the skin. Although its texture is hard, its surface is smooth after processing, making it very suitable for facial *gua sha*.

Jade facial *gua sha* scraper. A jade scraper dedicated to facial *gua sha*. The plane and edges are smooth. The four sides have different shapes. The curved radians of the corners are designed according to the curves of the different parts of the face. The short arc side is suitable for scraping the forehead, the long arc side is suitable for scraping the cheeks, and the two corners are suitable for scraping the acupoints around the eyes, the jaw, and the bridge of the nose. When in use, choose different parts of the scraper according to the curves and radians of the different parts of the face.

Jade facial *gua sha* scraper for eyes. This scraper is long and thin, with two symmetrical shallow and short arc sides and symmetrical long arc sides. The corner of the shallow and short arc is suitable for scraping the Jingming acupoint on the eyes, and the arc of the short side is suitable for laying flat on the Yuyao and Chengqi acupoints on the upper and lower eye sockets. When scraping the two points, the width of the short curved edges can effectively stimulate the scraped acupoints without causing pressure on the eyeballs, and the length of the tool is suitable for finger grip, making it easy to operate.

Jade *gua sha* scraper for body. This tool is rectangular, with smooth edges and rounded corners. The two long sides can scrape the holographic acupoints and meridian acupoints on the flat parts of the body. One short side of the tool has two symmetrical half-rounded corners. In addition to being suitable for scraping concave areas of the body, the two corners are especially suitable for scraping holographic acupoints on the spine, fingers, and head.

Scraping comb. Based on the original shape of the holographic meridian jade scraper, one long side is designed and processed into a thick, round, and blunt comb shape, which is convenient for combing the meridian points on the head, allowing for a

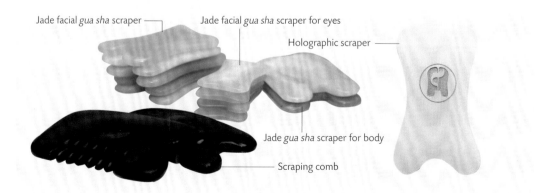

Jade facial *gua sha* scraper ——

Jade facial *gua sha* scraper for eyes

Holographic scraper ——

Jade *gua sha* scraper for body

Scraping comb

Fig. 10 Always use professional-grade tools for scraping, as it protects the skin while stimulating the meridian acupoints more effectively, leading to better results.

degree of pressure without hurting the head skin. As well as functioning as a scraper, the multi-functional holographic meridian comb is suitable for dredging the meridians of the head.

Holographic scraper. This delicate little jade scraper is suitable for scraping the second and third metacarpal bones of the hand. It can carry out precise three-dimensional positioning diagnosis and regulation of organs, viscera, and spine by scraping between the metacarpal bones.

Scraping oil. Scraping oil is processed with Chinese medicines with the function of clearing heat and detoxification, activating blood circulation and removing blood stasis, anti-inflammatory and analgesic without toxic side effects, or vegetable oils with strong permeability and good lubrication. The therapeutic effect of TCM helps to dredge the meridians, promote an impeded flow of *qi* and blood, promote blood circulation, and remove blood stasis. Vegetable oil has the function of moisturizing and protecting the skin. If TCM scraping oil is not available, you can use basic plant essential oils instead, or non-irritating moisturizing oils and lotions. Applying oil during scraping relieves pain, accelerates the expulsion of pathogenic factors, protects the skin, and prevents infection, making the facial *gua sha* safe and effective.

Facial *gua sha* cream. Facial scraping requires a lot of lubricant. If used on the face, liquid scraping oil will flow into the eyes or down the cheeks to the neck, so a special facial *gua sha* cream is used instead. It has good permeability and lubricity, and will not drip.

Make sure you choose scraping oil and cream that are non-irritant, free of dark pigments, and do not contain active ingredients for purposes such as softening the cuticles. Their only functions should be nourishing and hydrating.

Maintenance of Facial *Gua Sha* Tools

Jade scrapers can be washed and dried with soap or disinfected with ethanol. Jade scrapers are not prone to soaking or dryness, but bumps during storage should be avoided. In particular, scrapers should be used exclusively. This allows for easy portability and convenient *gua sha* sessions. It also helps to avoid cross-infection.

Cleansing Products

Towel or wet paper towel: It is best to use a towel or wet paper towel made of natural cellulose for cleansing before scraping.

Facial cleanser: The skin on the face should be cleaned before scraping. Makeup must be removed, and the skin should be cleaned with warm water or facial cleanser. Choose a facial cleanser that does not contain softening agents. The stratum corneum has a protective effect on the skin, so softening or removing it can leave skin unprotected. In winter, soak your jade scraper in hot water to warm it up first, bringing it close to skin temperature for increased comfort.

Scraping Techniques

The scraping techniques in this section include methods for facial *gua sha* and other parts of the body. Facial *gua sha* is different from body *gua sha* because the meridian must be unblocked for cosmetic treatment, and a certain amount of pressure is required, but it should not produce *sha*, which can affect aesthetics. The facial skin is sensitive to pain, and the person being scraped should not feel obvious pain during treatment. Therefore, the scraping speed must be uniform and slow, the pressure should be kept stable, and the scraping angle should be very small. These are the characteristics of the method dedicated to facial diagnosis, treatment, and beauty.

At the same time, facial *gua sha* requires not only scraping the face, but also other parts of the body, so as to treat both symptoms and root causes, and consolidate the beautifying effect of facial *gua sha*. Methods of flat-scraping, pushing and scraping, kneading and scraping, flat-pressing and kneading, vertical-pressing and kneading are also suitable for scraping other parts of the body. In addition, several special scraping methods are commonly used on other parts of the body.

Methods for Facial *Gua Sha*

1. Flat-pressing and kneading. Use the plane of the corner of the scraper to press on the acupoints at an angle of less than 15 degrees, and make slow and gentle rotating movements, keeping the plane of the corner of the scraper on the skin it touches. The points of force at the corners of the scraper, the pads of the fingers on the scraper, and the acupoints under the scraper are in a line. The pressing and kneading pressure should penetrate the subcutaneous tissue or muscle. Flat-pressing and kneading are used for the treatment and health care of key acupoints and holographic acupoint areas on the face.

2. Vertical-pressing and kneading. Press the corners of the tool on the acupoints at an angle of 90 degrees. The scraper should never leave the skin it touches. Make soft left-and-right, up-and-down, and slow intradermal pressing and kneading movements. This method is only used for scraping the Jingming acupoint on the face.

3. Flat-scraping. Hold the scraper, touch the skin with the edge of it, inclined in the direction of scraping, at an angle of less than 15 degrees. Scrape in a straight line in the same direction evenly and slowly, according to the needs of the scraping site, to a length of 3 to 5 centimeters, or 5 to 10 centimeters. It is advisable to scrape 2 to 3 times within one calm breath. Depending on the purpose and requirements of the scraping,

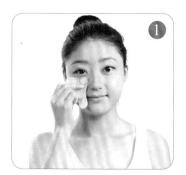 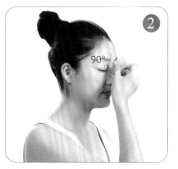 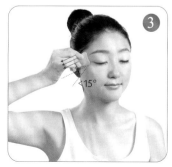

the pressure should penetrate the skin, above the muscle or above the bone, or into the muscle respectively. Flat-scraping method is used for facial skin care, and it is mostly applied at the beginning of facial *gua sha* and daily health care.

4. **Kneading and scraping.** Hold the scraper, and according to the size of the scraping area, touch the skin with one side edge of the scraper and the whole plane or half plane. Incline the scraper in the direction of scraping, and work evenly and continuously from the inside to the outside. Make slow, gentle rotations and scrape in an arc, that is, use the edge of one side of the scraper and the plane to rotate slowly. Move in an arc, and scrape while rubbing. Kneading and scraping method is used to dredge meridians, open up stasis points, and soothe and relax facial muscle stiffness and spasm.

5. **Pushing and scraping.** Hold the scraper, and touch the skin with the entire short side. Incline the scraper to the scraping direction at an angle of less than 15 degrees, and scrape in a straight line in the same direction evenly. The length of each scrape should be about 1 centimeter. It is advisable to scrape 2 to 3 times within one calm breath. The distance of each scrape is shorter than the flat-scraping method, but the speed is slower. The pressure penetrates the muscles and above the bones. The pushing and scraping method can find and eliminate positive reactions, and it is used for facial diagnosis and treatments for whitening and freckle removal.

6. **Rubbing and scraping.** Hold the scraper, and place the flat surface on the palm or the four fingers. Keep the fingers away from the skin, but keep the scraper close to it. Press the flat surface of the scraper with the force of the palm or four fingers. Penetrating the deep part of the facial muscles, the scraper can be evenly and continuously moved slowly and gently in an arc from bottom to top or from the outside to the inside. That is, while pressing, slowly rotate and move along the arc. Rubbing and scraping method is usually applied after scraping for facial diagnosis and treatment. The purpose is to dredge the blood circulation in the deep muscles and improve the blood supply to the whole face from the inside to the outside.

7. **Lifting.** Hold the scraper, and touch the skin with the entire long side (the short side can also be used for one-handed scraping by yourself). Incline the scraper in the direction of scraping, at an angle of 15 to 20 degrees. Scrape upwards from the bottom. The pressing force penetrates the deep part of the muscle, and lifts upwards. While scraping, the skin is lifted upwards with the muscle movement. Lifting method is mostly used after the scraping treatment, to perform overall facial lifting or scraping for lifting and thinning the face.

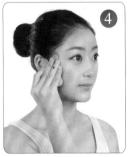 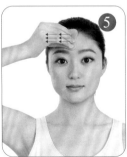 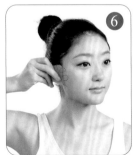 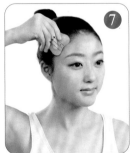

Scraping Methods for Other Parts of the Body

1. Surface-scraping. This is the most basic and commonly used method of scraping. Hold the scraper in your hand, and touch the skin with half of the long side or the whole long side, based on the need of the part. Tilt the scraper in the direction of scraping, and scrape evenly in the same direction from top to bottom or from the inside to the outside. Do not scrape back and forth. There must be a certain length of scraping each time. The angle of inclination of the scraper is based on the principle that it cannot only reduce pain for the patient, but also make it easier for the scraper to operate. Generally, the inclination is 30 to 60 degrees. The most widely used angle is 45 degrees. This scraping method is suitable for meridians and acupuncture points on relatively flat parts of the body, such as the torso, limbs, and flat parts of the head.

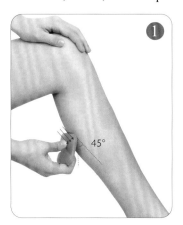
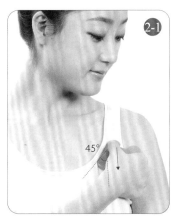
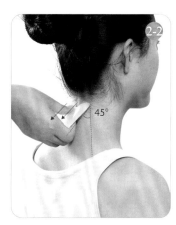

2. Angle-scraping (single angle-scraping, dual angle-scraping). In single angle-scraping, one corner of the scraper is used to scrape the acupoints from top to bottom, with the scraper inclined at 45 degrees to the scraping direction. This method is mostly used for the Jianzhen acupoint on the shoulder, the Danzhong and Zhongfu acupoints on the chest, and the Fengchi acupoint on the neck.

Dual angle-scraping uses the two corners of the groove of the scraper to scrape, aligning the groove with the spinous ridge, and placing the double angles on both sides of the groove between the spinous ridge and the transverse process on both sides. The scraper is tilted downward at 45 degrees, scraping from top to bottom. This scraping method is commonly used in the diagnosis, health care, and treatment of the spinal region.

3. Concentrated pressing. Place the corner of the scraper at a 90-degree angle perpendicular to the acupoints and press down, gradually increasing the force. Lift up quickly after a while to restore the muscles. Repeat this for many times. This scraping method is suitable for boneless soft tissue and bone gaps, and depressions such as the Renzhong acupoint.

4. Clapping. Bend the five fingers and the palm of the hand into an arc and clap. This method is mostly used on the meridian points of the limbs, especially the elbow pit and the knee pit. When the curved fingers and palms are in complete contact with the skin of the elbow and knee pits, this is called a full clap. When the curvature of the

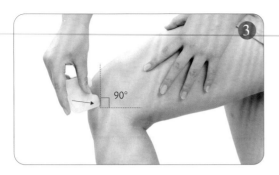
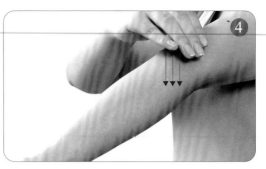

fingers and palms increases, and the two ends of the fingers and palms touch the inner and outer sides of the elbow and knee pits, and the middle of the palm does not touch the skin, this is called an empty clap. The effect of empty clapping is the same as that of full clapping; the difference is that empty clapping can relieve pain.

Clapping method has the same effect as the surface-scraping method, but produces *sha* quickly, and should only be applied to suitable candidates. It is not suitable for people with blood conditions or bleeding disorders, those taking anticoagulant drugs, and people with severe cardiovascular and cerebrovascular conditions. When clapping, be sure to apply scraping oil on the treatment area first. Clapping method is limited to the elbow and knee pits of the four limbs, and is prohibited in other parts. Clapping the elbow pit can treat and prevent upper limb pain, numbness, and heart and lung conditions; clapping the knee pit can treat and prevent lower limb pain, numbness, lower back pain, and neck pain.

5. Sharp-edge scraping. Put the corner of the scraper at a 90-degree angle perpendicular to the acupoint area without leaving the skin, and apply a certain amount of pressure to rub back and forth or left and right for a short distance (about 1 to 2 centimeters long). This method is suitable for the holographic acupoint area of the head. The area of the holographic acupoints on the head is small, requiring a lot of pressure for scraping. The scraper can move back and forth or left and right in the acupoints area.

6. Dredging meridians and *qi*. Use the long side of the scraper to scrape along the meridian from bottom to top or from top to bottom, using gentle, even, steady, and continuous force. The scraping surface should be long, generally from the elbow and knee joints to the tips of fingers and toes. This method is often used in *gua sha* treatment, after completing each segment of scraping, as well as during health care *gua sha* for overall meridian dredging, relaxing muscles, and eliminating fatigue.

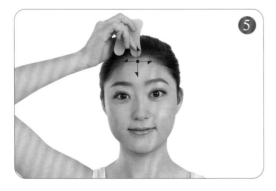
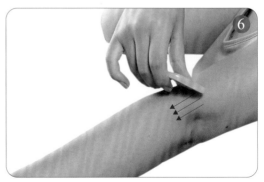

Different Scraping Methods for Different Parts of the Face

Facial features and skin condition are not only the characteristic signs of a person, but also reflect the health of their body. Complex and diverse skin problems occur on the face, and the same issue can appear in different areas, with completely different meanings. Therefore, when conducting facial *gua sha*, it is necessary to master the method of scraping different regions of the face, and understand the relationship between skin problems in different areas and the health of the body. Scraping the face can also regulate the corresponding parts of the body to consolidate the effects of cosmetic improvement.

Starting from the forehead at the top of the face and down to the jaw, the face is divided into six areas: the forehead area, eye area, nasal area, cheek area, perioral area, and lower jaw area.

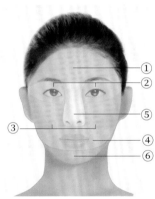

Fig. 11 Facial partition map.

① Forehead area: From the forehead to above the eyebrows, from the left and right to the hairline on both sides.
② Eye area: From the inner corner of the eye to the outer corner of the eye through the upper and lower orbits.
③ Cheek area: The middle part of the cheek from the lower eyelid to the underside of the cheekbone, from the side of the nose outward, up to the temple, down to the front of the ear.
④ Perioral area: The upper and lower sides of the mouth, from the outer corner of the mouth to the root of the ear.
⑤ Nasal area: From the base of the nose to the tip of the nose, from both sides of the base of the nose to wings of nose, and the nasal fossa.
⑥ Lower jaw area: From the middle of the lower jaw up to the Chengjiang acupoint, down to the Lianquan acupoint, and outside to the mandibular angle.

Self-Scraping

According to the division of the scraping area, the operation requirements, and the sequence, location, and method, a one-handed scraper is used to scrape sequentially, first on one side, then the other side, while sitting or lying. In the following chapters, scraping steps with order number in purple indicate self-scraping.

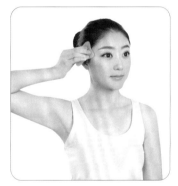

Scraping for Others

1. Take a lying position, and scrape the skin using the same partitions, methods, and sequence as in self-scraping.

2. First, hold the scraper in one hand and scrape the acupoints at the starting point of each area in the middle of the face in sequence according to the steps.

3. Then, hold a scraper in each hand, and scrape from the middle to both sides at the same time.

In the following chapters, scraping steps with order number in pink indicate scraping for others.

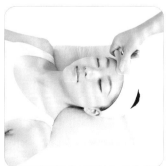

Scraping Methods for the Forehead Area

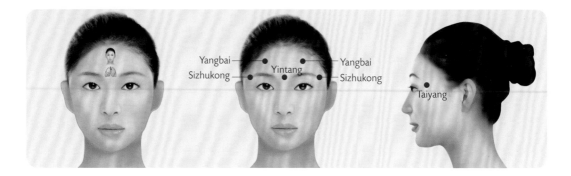

Yangbai — Yintang — Yangbai
Sizhukong — Sizhukong
Taiyang

1. Scrape the upper forehead area first, press and knead the head area with the flat-pressing and kneading method with the corner of the scraper.

    2. Use the short arc edge of the scraper to scrape from the middle of the forehead to both sides to the temples with the flat-scraping method.

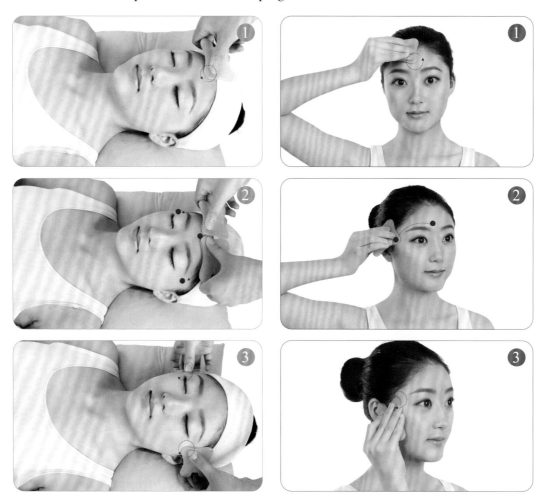

* Most of the steps in the book show both scraping on others (pink) and self-scraping (purple) at the same time.

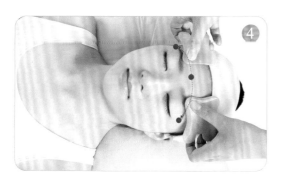
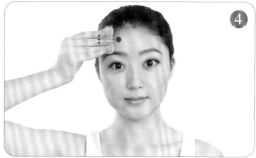

3. Press and knead the Taiyang acupoints with the flat-pressing and kneading method with the corner of the scraper.

4. Use the flat-pressing and kneading method to press and knead the throat area at the lower frontal region, then scrape from the throat area at the forehead region outwards to the Taiyang acupoints on both sides through the Cuanzhu, Yangbai, and Sizhukong acupoints.

Scraping Methods for the Eye Area

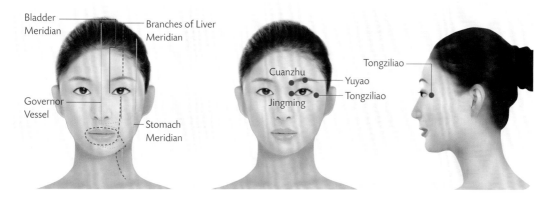

1. Press and knead the Jingming point with the vertical-pressing and kneading method.

2. Scrape from the Jingming acupoint along the edge of the upper orbital bone and pass through the Liver Meridian to the Tongziliao acupoint at the outer corner of the eye.

3. Press and knead the Tongziliao point with the flat-pressing and kneading method with the corners of facial *gua sha* scraper or *gua sha* scraper for eyes.

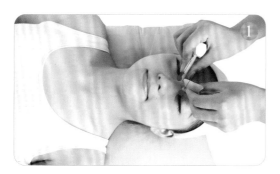
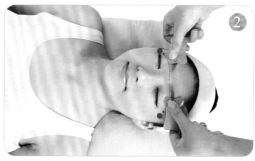

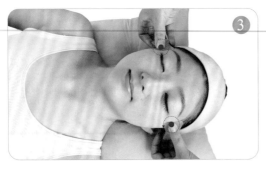
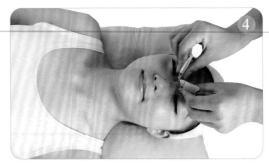

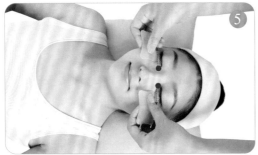
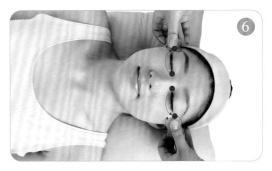

4. Then scrape the lower eye socket area. First, use the corner of the facial *gua sha* scraper or *gua sha* scraper for eyes to press and knead the Jingming acupoint with the vertical-pressing and kneading method.

5. Use the long curved edge of the scraper to flat-scrape from the Jingming acupoint along the edge of the lower orbital bone outward, through the Liver Meridian to the Tongziliao acupoint at the outer corner of the eye.

6. Press and knead the Tongziliao acupoint with the flat-pressing and kneading method with the corners of the facial *gua sha* scraper or *gua sha* scraper for eyes.

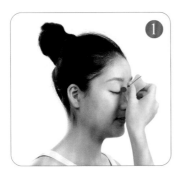
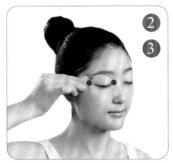
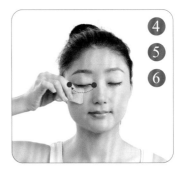

Scraping Methods for the Cheek Area

1. Scrape the upper cheek area first, press and knead the Shangyingxiang acupoint with the corner of the facial *gua sha* scraper using the flat-pressing and kneading method.

2. Scrape from the Shangyingxiang acupoint through the Chengqi and Sibai acupoints, and the upper limbs area outward and upward to the Taiyang acupoints.

3. Use the corner of the facial *gua sha* scraper to press and knead the Taiyang acupoints with the flat-pressing and kneading method.

4. Then scrape the lower cheek area, press and knead the Yingxiang acupoint with the corner of the facial *gua sha* scraper using the flat-pressing and kneading method.

5. Using the long-curved edge of the tool,

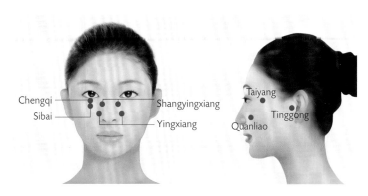

Chengqi
Sibai
Shangyingxiang
Yingxiang
Taiyang
Tinggong
Quanliao

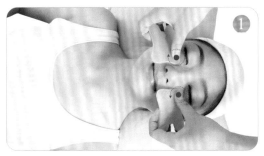

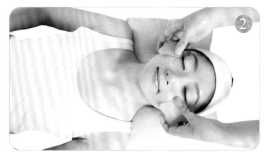

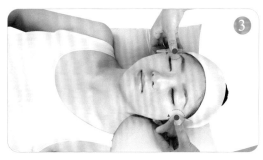

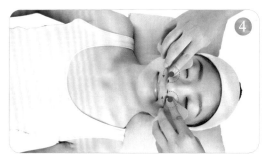

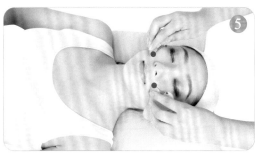

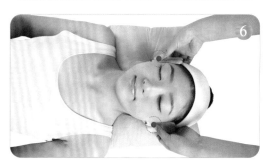

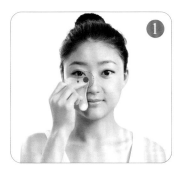

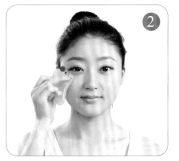

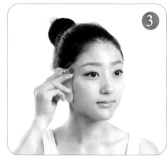

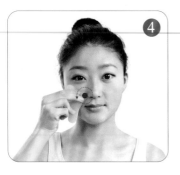
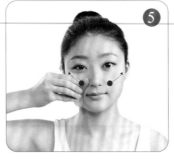
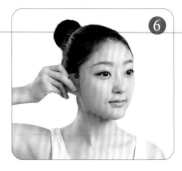

scrape from the Yingxiang acupoint upward along the inner and lower cheekbones via the Quanliao acupoint with the flat-scraping method.

6. Press and knead the Tinggong acupoint with the flat-pressing and kneading method using the corner of the facial *gua sha* scraper.

Scraping Methods for the Perioral Area

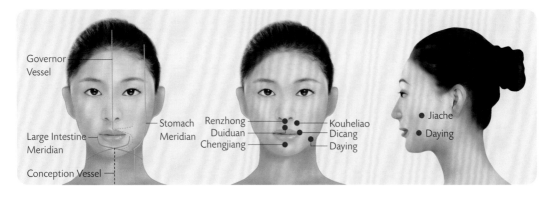

1. Scrape the upper part of the lips first, press and knead the Renzhong acupoint with the flat-pressing and kneading method using the corner of the facial *gua sha* scraper.

2. Use the flat-scraping method to scrape from the Renzhong and Duiduan acupoints of the nasolabial fold along the skin of the upper lip through the Kouheliao acupoint on both sides to the Dicang acupoint at the corner of the mouth.

3. Press and knead the Dicang acupoint with the flat-pressing and kneading method using the corner of the facial *gua sha* scraper.

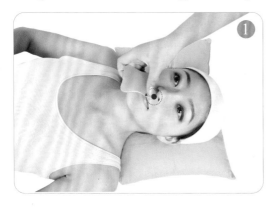
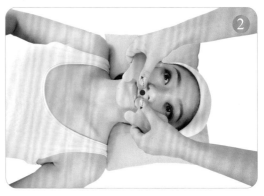

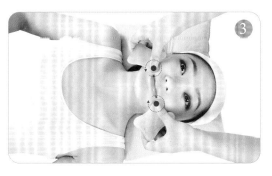 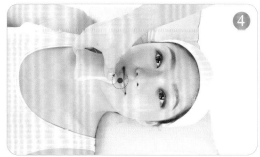

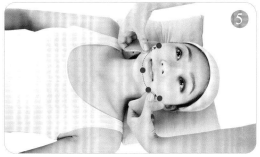 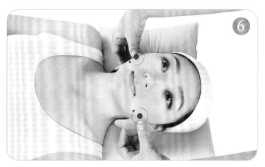

4. Scrape the lower part of the lips, press and knead the Chengjiang acupoint with the flat-pressing and kneading method using the corner of the facial *gua sha* scraper.

5. Use the flat-scraping method to scrape along the Stomach Meridian from the Chengjiang acupoint, through Dicang acupoint, Daying acupoint, and the lower limb area, outwards and upwards to the Jiache acupoint.

6. Press and knead the Jiache acupoint with the flat-pressing and kneading method.

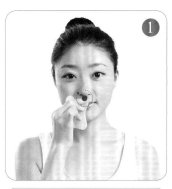 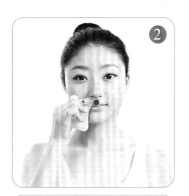 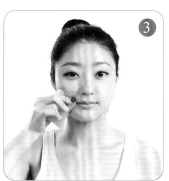

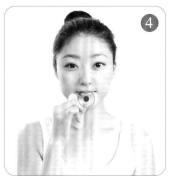 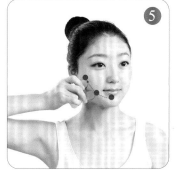 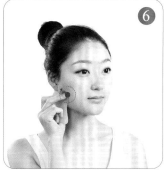

Scraping Methods for the Nosal Area

1. Scrape the middle of the nose first, using the long arc of the facial *gua sha* scraper to scrape the heart area from the root of the nose between the eyes, and the liver area in the middle of the nose bridge, to the spleen area at the tip of the nose.

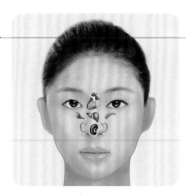

2. Then, scrape both sides of the nose, using the two corners of the facial *gua sha* scraper to ride the bridge of the nose, and using the flat-scraping method to scrape

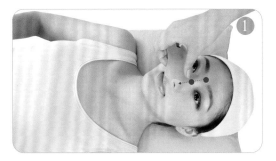

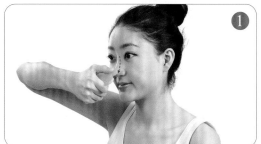

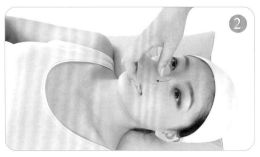

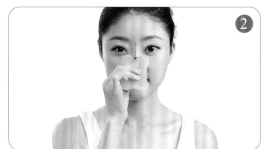

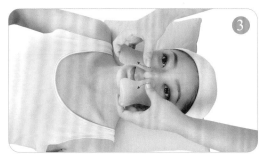

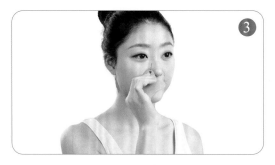

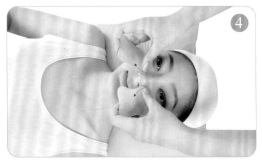

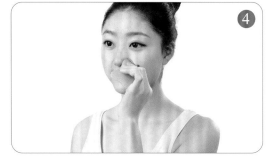

from the root of the nose through the gallbladder area and pancreas area to the stomach area on the wings of nose.

3. You can also use the corner of the facial *gua sha* scraper to scrape the gallbladder area, pancreas area, and stomach area respectively with the flat-scraping method.

4. Use the corner of the facial *gua sha* scraper to scrape the nasal fossa from top to inner bottom.

Scraping Methods for the Lower Jaw Area

1. Scrape the middle of the lower jaw first, using the groove in the middle of the two corners of the facial *gua sha* scraper to straddle the middle of the lower jaw; use flat-scraping method to scrape the Conception Vessel area.

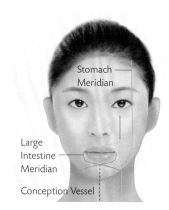

2. Use the flat-scraping method with the corner groove of the facial *gua sha* scraper to scrape from the middle of the lower jaw to the angle of mandible on both sides.

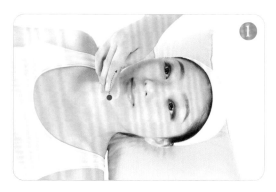
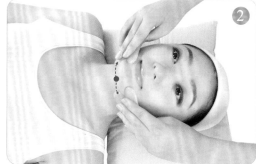

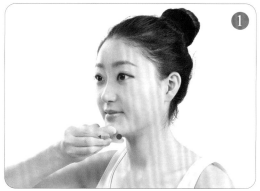
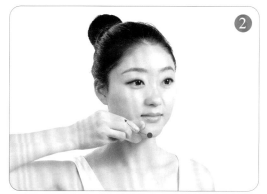

CHAPTER THREE
Gua Sha for Daily Beauty

Holographic meridian facial *gua sha* offers health care and diagnosis as well as cosmetic improvement. It can be used to check the meridians, viscera, and organs for sub-health in the body, and can macroscopically judge the degree and nature of sub-health, identifying related factors that affect the facial appearance.

Facial scraping for whitening, chloasma removal, skin rejuvenation, wrinkles removal, face thinning, and skin firming all require different techniques. For different purposes of each type of scraping, there are obvious differences in the pressure of the scraper, the depth of penetration into the skin, the method of scraping, and the speed and direction of the force. This chapter will explain the various techniques of facial *gua sha* for different types of cosmetic improvement. If you understand them and practice them carefully, you will achieve good beautifying effects.

A standard, complete facial scraping operation should be divided into four steps: lubricating the skin and removing wrinkles, diagnosing health, whitening and removing chloasma, and firming the skin and slimming the face. For personal facial *gua sha* at home, you can follow the order of this chapter, or you can choose one of the steps to work according to your own situation and needs.

Note: Some acupoints involved in this book are distributed symmetrically on both sides of the body. When conducting facial *gua sha*, except for a few acupoints that require one-sided scraping, the rest are all symmetrical acupoints on both sides of the body by default.

Preparation

Before scraping, clean the face with warm water, then apply facial *gua sha* cream. If you have the right conditions, follow the method below and the results will be better. Remember that the most important thing is to apply a sufficient amount of facial *gua sha* cream to ensure sufficient lubrication during scraping.

1. First, wrap the hair along the hairline with a soft clean towel.

2. Apply a warm clean towel to the face for 3 minutes before scraping, for comfort.

3. Squeeze out a peanut-sized portion of facial *gua sha* cream onto the forehead, nose tip, both cheeks, and lower jaw, in that order.

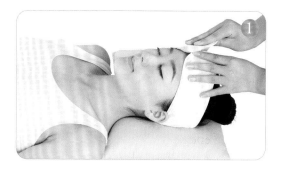

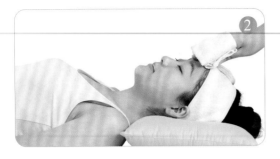

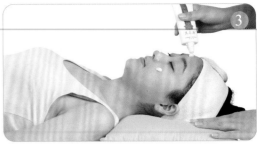

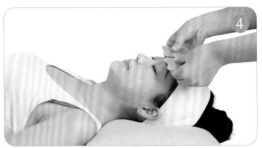

4. Spread the facial *gua sha* cream evenly with your hands or a facial *gua sha* scraper over the entire face, and start scraping. In winter, you can soak the facial *gua sha* scraper in warm water at about 50°C for 10 minutes before starting to scrape.

Scraping for Lubricating Skin and Removing Wrinkles

If you are performing facial *gua sha* for the first time, the lubricating and wrinkle-removing method is a good place to start. The pressure is relatively light, and only penetrates the soft tissue under the skin and above the muscle. The purpose is to unblock the meridians of the skin and subcutaneous tissue, improve the microcirculation of the dermis, stimulate the skin cells, and promote skin metabolism, which can improve the nutrient supply of the skin, activate cells, relieve wrinkles, improve a sallow complexion, add luster, rejuvenate the complexion, shrink pores, refine the skin, and delay skin aging.

Key Points of the Technique

1. The scraping method must be gentle and slow. The pressure penetrates the soft tissue under the skin and above the muscles. Don't scrape the surface of the skin without any pressure. Nor should the pressure be so strong that it penetrates deep into the muscles and bones.

2. Scrape from top to bottom. Scrape the forehead, eye area, cheeks, mouth area, nose, and lower jaw area in sequence according to the different *gua sha* methods for different parts of the face. According to the operation requirements of this method, the sequence is from the inside to the outside, along the muscle texture and bone shape, focusing on the parts that are prone to wrinkles.

3. When scraping, start each area with a scraper holding in one hand. Press and knead the middle acupoint area of the face (except the nose). Use the flat-scraping method to work directly from the starting point of the acupoint area (except the Jingming acupoint and nose area) to the end point of the acupoint area without stopping in the middle, and end with the flat-pressing and kneading method at the end point of each scraping.

4. The scraping speed is no more than 3 times within one calm breath. Scrape 5 to 10 times on each point or part.

5. When scraping for others, hold a scraper in each hand and scrape the left and right sides at the same time. For self-scraping at home, you can hold the scraper with one hand, scrape one side of the face, and then the other side.

Recommended Procedures

1. To maintain the skin of the forehead area and reduce wrinkles: First scrape the upper forehead area, use the corner of the the facial *gua sha* scraper to press and knead the head area with flat-pressing and kneading method. Use the short arc of the scraper to scrape from the middle of the forehead to both sides towards the Taiyang acupoints with the flat-scraping method. Press and knead the Taiyang acupoints with the flat-pressing and kneading method with the corners of the scraper. Then use the same method to scrape every acupoint or part above the lower forehead area, for 5 to 10 times each time.

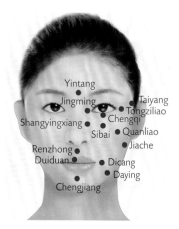

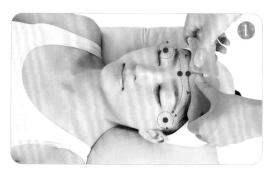

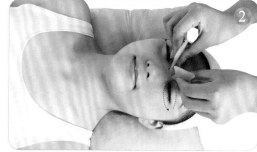

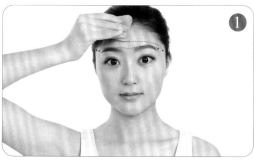

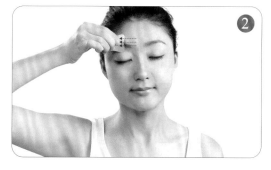

2. To maintain the skin around the eyes and reduce wrinkles: First scrape the upper eye socket area. Use the corner of the facial *gua sha* scraper or scraper for eyes to press and knead the Jingming acupoint with the vertical-pressing and kneading method; use the flat-scraping method with the upper end of the long arc of the facial *gua sha* scraper or with the short arc of the facial *gua sha* scraper for eyes to scrape from the Jingming acupoint along the upper eye socket and out through the Liver Meridian to the Tongziliao acupoint at the outer corner of the eye. Use the corner of the facial *gua sha* scraper or scraper for eyes to press and knead the Tongziliao acupoint with the flat-pressing and kneading method. Scrape the lower orbital area in the same way.

   3. **To maintain the skin of the cheek area and reduce wrinkles:** First scrape the upper cheek area, and use the flat-pressing and kneading method to press and knead the Shangyingxiang acupoint with the corner of the facial *gua sha* scraper. Use the long arc of the scraper to scrape from the Shangyingxiang acupoint along the Chengqi acupoint, Sibai acupoint, and the upper limb area to the Taiyang acupoints with the flat-scraping method. Press and knead the Taiyang acupoints with the flat-pressing and kneading method using the corner of the scraper.

   Then scrape the lower cheek area, and press and knead the Yingxiang acupoint with the flat-pressing and kneading method using the corner of the facial *gua sha* scraper. Use the long arc of the scraper to scrape from the Yingxiang acupoint along the inner and lower side of the cheekbones via the Quanliao acupoint to the Tinggong acupoint with the flat-scraping method. Press and knead the Tinggong acupoint with the flat-pressing and kneading method using the corner of the scraper.

   4. **To maintain the skin of the perioral area and reduce wrinkles:** First scrape the upper part of the lips. Press and knead the Renzhong acupoint with the flat-pressing and kneading method, then use the flat-scraping method to scrape from the Renzhong acupoint and the Duiduan acupoint along the skin of the upper lip through the Heliao acupoint to the Dicang acupoint. Press and knead the Dicang acupoint with the corner of the scraper using the flat-pressing and kneading method. Press and knead the Chengjiang acupoint using flat-pressing and kneading method and then scrape the lower part of the lips. Scrape along the Stomach Meridian from the Chengjiang acupoint through the

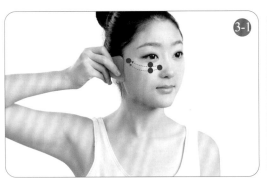

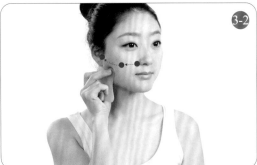

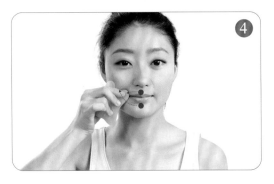

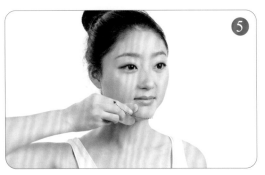

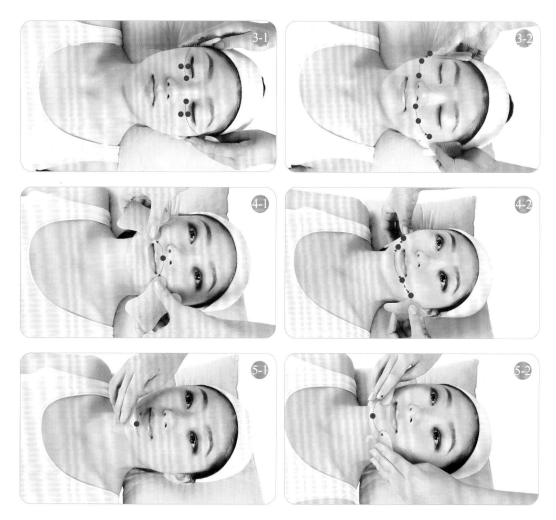

Dicang acupoint, and the Daying acupoint to the Jiache acupoint with the flat-scraping method. Press and knead the Jiache acupoint with the flat-pressing and kneading method.

    5. To maintain the skin of the lower jaw area and reduce wrinkles: First scrape the middle of the lower jaw. Use the groove between the two corners of the facial *gua sha* scraper to straddle the middle of the lower jaw bone, and scrape the Conception Vessel area with the flat-scraping method. Then scrape from the middle of the lower jaw to both sides to the angle of mandible using the flat-scraping method with the corner groove of the scraper.

Scraping for Diagnosing Health

During the scraping process, focus on finding the positive reactions, that is, scrape the parts that offer resistance. You can judge the sub-health of the viscera and organs according to the meridians, acupoints, and holographic acupoints where the positive reaction parts belong, as well as the reasons for their problems. With any slight changes in the body, no matter whether there are physical symptoms or not, there will be different degrees of positive reactions in the facial connected meridians and corresponding viscera and organ acupoints. There will also be different degrees of positive reactions under abnormal skin tone and melasma, such as astringent skin, subcutaneous gravel, nodules, pain, muscle tension, stiffness, and fibrous bands. The location, depth, nature, and morphological characteristics of these positive reactions can point out the cause and nature of abnormal skin color. Referring to the above-mentioned diagnostic rules of positive reactions (pages 26 to 27), you can quickly identify the location and degree of sub-health in the body.

The scraping method for diagnosing health also has the effect of dredging meridians, opening *xuan fu*, and improving microcirculation. Therefore, while identifying the cause of unsightly skin conditions, it also has the effects of stimulating skin cell vitality, promoting metabolism, and improving abnormal skin tone to varying degrees.

Key Points of the Technique

1. The pressure of scraping and pressing should penetrate the layers of tissue under the skin, in the muscle, and above the bone, checking whether there is a positive reaction in each layer of tissue. Do not use too much pressure, as it penetrates the bone, which is not conducive to finding a positive reaction.

2. The whole process of facial *gua sha* is performed by pushing and scraping method (except for the Jingming acupoint), and the scraping distance should be short, advancing by 1 centimeter each time. For those with dark circles, to eliminate the positive reaction on the Bladder Meridian between the Jingming acupoint and Cuanzhu acupoint, it is necessary to push and scrape, advancing by 1 millimeter at a time. The scraping speed should be controlled to scrape 1 to 2 times within one calm breath. Since each acupoint area or acupoint range is small, the positive reaction is like fine sand and gravel, and the skin will feel slightly astringent, it is necessary to search 1 centimeter by 1 centimeter carefully, and feel for abnormal changes under the scraper while scraping to identify whether there is any abnormality such as astringency, subcutaneous grit, nodules, pain response, and the nature of the pain, whether there is muscle tension and stiffness, looseness and weakness, bulging, or an empty feeling under the scraper. Each part needs to be scraped 5 to 10 times.

3. Each part is first pushed and scraped from the middle acupoint area of the face with a scraper holding in one hand. According to the operation requirements and sequence of the different *gua sha* methods for different parts of the face, scrape from the inside to the outside along with the muscle texture and bone shape, focusing on scraping the meridian circulating parts, acupoints, and holographic acupoints.

4. Use the vertical-pressing and kneading method with the corner of the facial *gua sha* scraper for eyes to diagnose the Jingming acupoint. Use the corner of the scraper to press vertically on the Jingming acupoint. The pressure gradually penetrates above the bone without leaving the skin. Perform slow massage on the skin. Go up and down and side to side to look for positive reactions in the subcutaneous soft tissue.

5. Areas with chloasma and abnormal color, such as dark circles, eye bags, and dark

areas should be scraped with emphahsis.

6. When scraping for others, hold a scraper in each hand and scrape the left and right sides at the same time. For self-scraping at home, you can hold the scraper with one hand, scrape one side of the face, and then scrape the other side.

Recommended Procedures
1. Diagnosing the forehead area: Push and scrape the head area, push and scrape the central Governor Vessel and Bladder Meridian from the inside to the outside, push and scrape the Yangbai acupoint, the throat area, and the Sizhukong acupoint, and push and scrape the Taiyang acupoints from the inside out to the top.

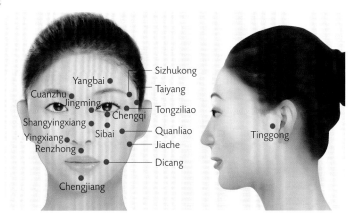

2. Diagnosing the eye area: Press and knead the Jingming acupoint vertically, push and scrape the Bladder Meridian on both sides of the root of the nose from bottom to top, push and scrape the Cuanzhu acupoint, the Liver Meridian of the upper eye orbit, and the Liver Meridian of the lower eye orbit, and push and scrape the Tongziliao acupoint from the inside out to the top.

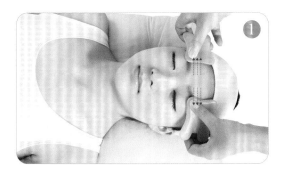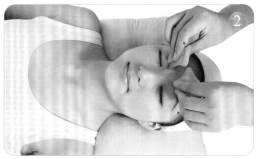

3. Diagnosing the nasal area: Push and scrape the lung area, heart area, liver area, gallbladder area, pancreas area, spleen area, stomach area, and nasal groove from top to bottom.

4. Diagnosing the cheek area: Push and scrape the Shangyingxiang acupoint from the inside out to the top; push and scrape the Chengqi acupoint, Sibai acupoint, upper limb area, and Yingxiang acupoint; push the Quanliao acupoint from the bottom to the top, and push and scrape the Tinggong acupoint from inside to outside.

5. Diagnosing the perioral area: Push and scrape the Renzhong acupoint; push and scrape the upper lip bladder area from inside to outside; push and scrape the Dicang

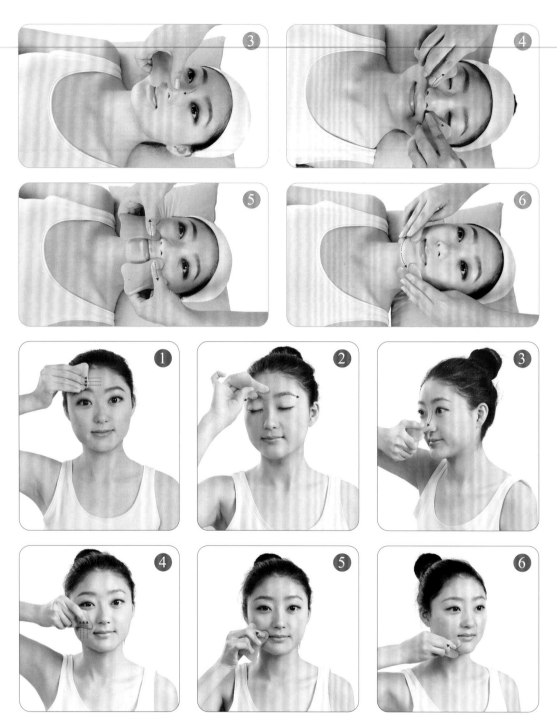

acupoint from bottom to top; push and scrape the Chengjiang acupoint; push and scrape the Stomach Meridian from inside out to the top; push and scrape the lower limb area, and the Jiache acupoint.

6. **Diagnosing the lower jaw area:** Push and scrape the Conception Vessel; push and scrape the mandibular area from inside to outside; push and scrape the Stomach Meridian, Large Intestine Meridian, and Small Intestine Meridian.

Scraping for Skin Whitening and Removing Chloasma

The whitening and chloasma-removing scraping method helps to lighten and eliminate dark spots, improve dark circles and yellowish and dull complexions, and make the complexion even and beautiful. The key to this method is to find the positive reactions, and improve the microcirculation of the dermis, subcutaneous fat, and muscle tissue through the scraping technique, gradually eliminating the positive reaction of the sallow complexion under the pigmentation, dullness, and dark circles. Positive reactions such as skin astringency, subcutaneous grit, nodules, pain, muscle tension, and stiffness are manifestations of *qi* and blood stasis in different tissue meridians. These positive reactions are products of *qi* and blood stagnation and further impede the operation of *qi* and blood, allowing local metabolites to accumulate and aggravating facial skin problems. Scraping to eliminate these positive reactions will stop this vicious cycle, clear the meridians, and give the skin sufficient *qi* and blood supply. The smooth meridians will gradually eliminate the metabolites, promote the decomposition of melanin, and restore the natural beauty of the skin. Therefore, the process of eliminating positive reactions is the process of whitening and lightening spots.

Key Points of the Technique

1. If you are trying facial *gua sha* for the first time, the whitening and chloasma-removing scraping method is best performed after the health-diagnosing scraping method, because only after this step can the location, degree, and nature of the positive reaction be known. Frequent practitioners of facial *gua sha* already know the positive reaction parts well, so they can move directly to whitening and chloasma-removing scraping.

2. The scraping method for whitening and chloasma-removing is selected according to the characteristics of positive reactions, including the pushing and scraping method, kneading and scraping method and flat-pressing and kneading method. The area of positive reactions is relatively large, such as areas with astringent skin, muscle tension and stiffness, or areas with more gravel nodules, as well as sensitive points and sensitive areas with severe pain, are suitable for the kneading and scraping method. For single, isolated gravel nodules, use pushing and scraping method or flat-pressing and kneading method.

3. For various scraping methods, the pressing force should be determined according to the depth of the positive reaction sites. Pressure should penetrate each layer of tissue under the skin, in the muscle, and above the bone where the positive reaction is located. Although eliminating positive reactions is the key to whitening and chloasma removal, it requires a process, and should not be rushed. Do not use too much pressure, as it will penetrate the bones, which is not conducive to finding a positive reaction.

4. Scrape the positive reactions of lower eyelid eye bags or dark circles with the flat-pressing and kneading method. Since the eyelid skin is the thinnest and most tender, avoid frequent scraping that loosens the skin. The Jingming acupoint is very sensitive, and the vertical-pressing and kneading pressure should penetrate above the bone gradually. The scraper should not leave the skin, and should slowly move up and down and left and right in the skin to eliminate the positive reaction in the

subcutaneous soft tissue.

5. Key points of using the pushing and scraping method to eliminate positive reactions: The scraping distance should be short, advancing 1 centimeter each time. For those with dark circles, to eliminate the positive reactions on the Bladder Meridian between the Jingming acupoint and Cuanzhu acupoint, it is necessary to push and scrape, advancing by 1 millimeter at a time. The scraping speed should be controlled to 1 to 2 times within one calm breath no matter for the push-scraping method, vertical-pressing and kneading method, or kneading and scraping method. For loose, weak muscles and areas with a feeling of emptiness under the scraper, the pressure should be reduced appropriately. Each part needs to be scraped 5 to 15 times.

6. Each part should be scraped from the middle acupoint of the face with a scraper holding in one hand, from top to bottom according to the sequence of the different *gua sha* methods for different parts of the face, from the forehead, around the eyes, the cheeks, around the mouth, nose, and jaw, from the inside to the outside (except for the nose); scrape along the muscle texture and bone shape. Areas without positive reactions can be ignored and not scraped. The focus of scraping should be parts with chloasma, abnormal shape and color, such as dark circles, bags under the eyes, and dull color.

7. When scraping for others, hold a scraper in each hand and scrape the left and right sides at the same time. For self-scraping at home, you can hold the scraper with one hand, scrape one side of the face, and then scrape the other side. Scrape each part 10 to 15 times depending on the severity of the positive reactions.

Recommended Procedures

1. Whitening and chloasma removal on the forehead:
Push and scrape the Yintang acupoint, knead and scrape the Gallbladder Meridian on the forehead, push and scrape the Yangbai acupoint from the inside out, knead and scrape the Taiyang acupoints, then push and scrape or knead and scrape the skin with stains and dullness.

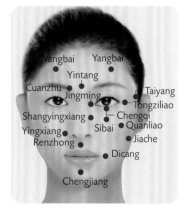

2. Whitening around the eyes, improving dark circles: Press and knead the Jingming acupoint vertically, push and scrape the Bladder Meridian next to the nose from bottom to top, push and scrape the Cuanzhu acupoint, push and scrape the Liver Meridian of the upper

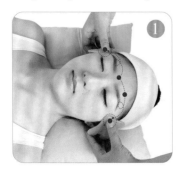
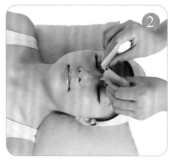
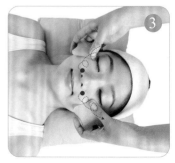

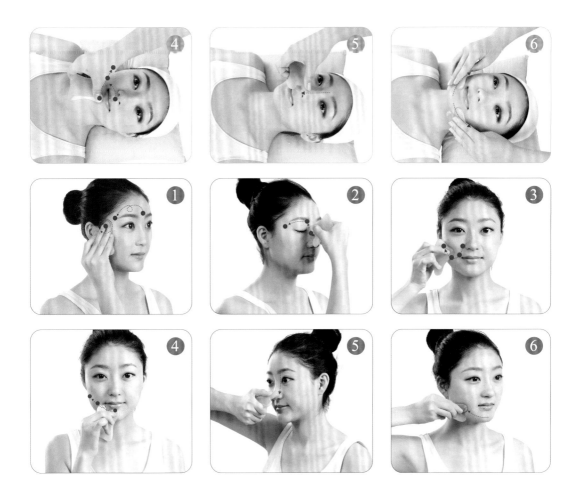

and lower orbits, and push and scrape the Tongziliao acupoint.

3. **Whitening and chloasma removal on the cheeks:** Push and scrape the Shangyingxiang acupoint from inside out and up, flat-press and knead the Chengqi and Sibai acupoints, knead and scrape the upper limb area, push and scrape the Yingxiang acupoint, push and scrape or knead and scrape the Quanliao acupoint; knead and scrape the lower limb area, then push and scrape or knead and scrape the skin with stains and dullness.

4. **Whitening and chloasma removal around the mouth:** Push and scrape the Renzhong acupoint, push and scrape the bladder area of the upper lip, push and scrape the Dicang acupoint from the bottom to the outside and up, push and scrape the Chengjiang acupoint, push and scrape the Stomach Meridian from the inside out and up, knead and scrape the Jiache acupoint, and push and scrape or knead and scrape the skin with stains and dullness.

5. **Whitening and chloasma removal in the nasal area:** Push and scrape the heart area from top to bottom, then push and scrape the liver area, gallbladder area, pancreas area, spleen area, and stomach area.

6. **Whitening and chloasma removal on the lower jaw:** Push and scrape the Conception Vessel, push and scrape the Stomach Meridian, Large Intestine Meridian, and Small Intestine Meridian in the lower jaw area from inside to outside.

Scraping for Firming the Skin and Slimming the Face

This scraping method helps to improve sagging skin, lift the corners of the eyes and mouth, restore muscle elasticity, and tighten the skin. The key is to use the rubbing and scraping method, and lifting method to scrape, press and knead the key acupoints, promoting lymphatic circulation and blood circulation, and unblocking the local meridians and the flow of *qi* and blood of meridian tendons in the meridian system, which can enhance the elasticity of muscle fibers and increase the flexibility of elastic fibers in the fascia. Through these fine adjustments, sagging skin can be transformed to lift, firm, and slim the face.

Key Points of the Technique

1. *Gua sha* for skin firming and face slimming is best performed after scraping for health diagnosis and treatment, because after these two steps, the positive reactions will have been found or eliminated to varying degrees, and the microcirculation of the skin and subcutaneous tissue will have been improved. On this basis, the scraping of key acupoints can firm and slim the face more effectively.

2. *Gua sha* for skin firming and face slimming involves the rubbing and scraping method and lifting method. The main point of these two scraping methods is that the plane of the scraper is close to the skin, and the pressure penetrates deep into the facial muscles. Both scraping methods can dredge the meridians in the deep part of the muscle, promote the *qi* and blood circulation in the tendons, restore the elasticity of the muscles, and improve the flexibility of the fascia.

3. The focus of lifting method and rubbing and scraping method is to identify the start and end acupoints of each step. The scraping technique for lifting and firming the skin involves paying attention to the direction of scraping, and always lifting and moving upward. The pressing force must penetrate the deep part of the muscle. The scraper should be close to the skin, and the area of contact is maximized. It is the movement of the scraper in the deeper part of the muscle that drives the movement of the skin. Avoid pulling the muscle along with the movement of the skin.

4. *Gua sha* for skin firming and face slimming is divided into two steps: relaxation and lifting. Scrape from the jaw up to the forehead. First use rubbing and scraping method to clear the meridians, increase blood flow, and increase muscle nutrition, and then use the lifting method to scrape.

5. If you have not performed the procedures of scraping for health diagnosis and treatment, and are performing the method for skin firming and slimming directly, for each operation mentioned above, you should first flat-press and knead the starting acupoint 5 times. The pressing force should penetrate the deep part of the muscle. Use this acupoint as the starting point again, and perform the rubbing and scraping method, and lifting in sequence, in an upward direction.

6. When using the rubbing and scraping method on others, hold a scraper in each hand and scrape the left and right sides at the same time. When performing the lifting

method on others, hold a scraper in each hand and put them on the same side of the face. Using the whole long side to touch the skin. The scrapers should be inclined in the direction of scraping, at an angle of inclination of 20 to 30 degrees. The two scrapers alternate from bottom to top. When self-scraping at home, you can hold the scraper with one hand, scrape one side of the face, and then scrape the other side.

Recommended Procedures

First, scrape the areas using the rubbing and scraping method. Scrape the jaw area, mouth corner area, inner cheek area, outer cheek area, outer eye corner area, and forehead area

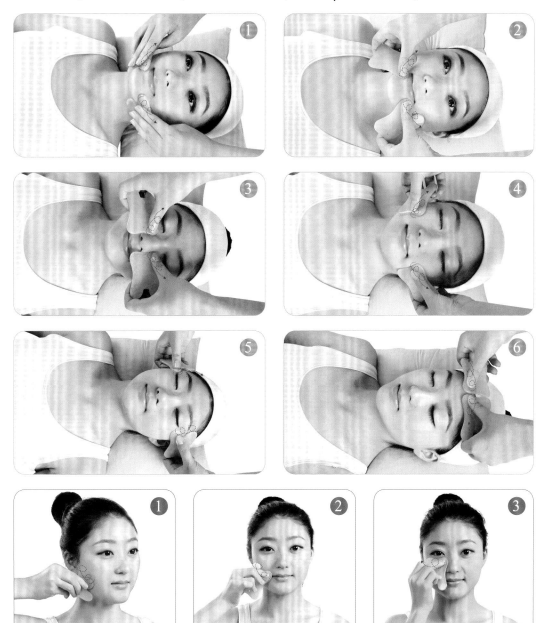

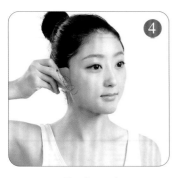

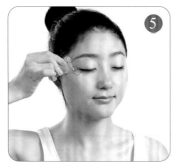

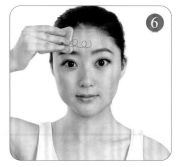

sequentially from bottom to top with the rubbing and scraping method, scraping each area 5 to 10 times.

The second step is to scrape each area with lifting method. After scraping each acupoint with the flat-pressing and kneading method, the acupoint is used as a starting point to scrape upwards with lifting. Details are as follows.

1. Lifting and firming the lower jaw: Flat-press and knead the Lianquan and Chengjiang acupoints in turn, 5 times for each point, then use the lifting method to scrape from the Lianquan and Chengjiang acupoints to the front of the ear respectively. Be sure to place the edge of the scraper on the skin between the Lianquan acupoint and the lower jaw, scrape from the middle of lower jaw outward to the angle of mandible, and then lift it up to the front of the ear. Scrape each part with the lifting method 5 to 10 times.

2. Lifting the corners of the mouth: Flat-press and knead the Renzhong, Chengjiang, and Dicang

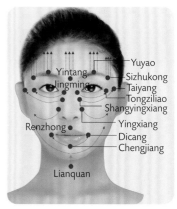

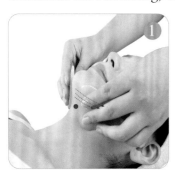

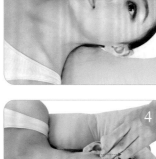

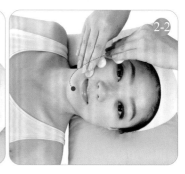

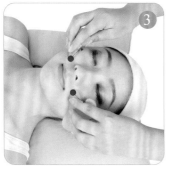

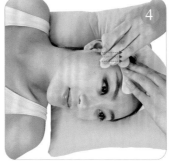

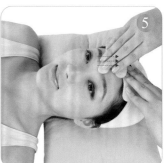

acupoints in turn, 5 times respectively. After pressing and kneading the acupoints, lift and scrape outwards and upwards to the top of the ear, 5 to 10 times for each part.

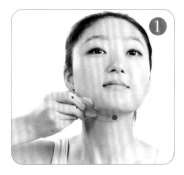 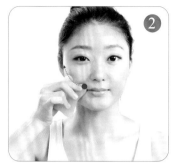

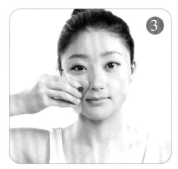 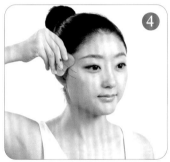 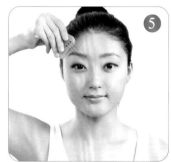

3. Slimming the face and lifting the cheeks: Flat-press and knead the Yingxiang, Quanliao, and Shangyingxiang acupoints, upper limb area, and Taiyang acupoint in turn, 5 times respectively. After that, lift and scrape outwards and upwards from the acupoints to the forehead hairline, 5 to 10 times for each acupoint.

4. Lifting the corners of the eyes: Flat-press and knead the Tongziliao, Taiyang and Sizhukong acupoints in turn, 5 times respectively. After pressing and kneading, lift and scrape from the acupoints to the forehead and hairline, 5 to 10 times respectively.

5. Lifting the forehead: Flat-press and knead the Yuyao and Yintang acupoints in turn, 5 times respectively. After pressing and kneading, lift and scrape from the acupoints to the anterior hairline, 5 to 10 times respectively.

Skin Care and Precautions after *Gua Sha*

1. Use a soft towel soaked in warm water or a wet tissue to clean the face in the order of the jaw, around the mouth, cheeks, nose, eye area, and forehead.

2. Pat moisturizing lotion on. If conditions permit, soak a small piece of facial tissue with conditioning lotion, and pat it onto the jaw, around the mouth, cheeks, nose, around the eyes, and forehead in that order.

3. If conditions permit, apply a heated nutritional mask after scraping, and keep it on for 15 minutes. At this time, the skin pores are slightly opened, and the subcutaneous blood circulation is strong, which is conducive to the absorption of nutrients.

4. Remove the mask and apply a moisturizing lotion or nourishing cream.

5. After facial *gua sha*, drink a cup of warm water and keep warm. In the winter, stay indoors for 30 minutes after the scraping session.

CHAPTER FOUR
Removing Dullness and Brightening the Skin

The bottom part of the epidermis of the skin is the basal layer (in addition to keratinocytes in the basal layer, there are melanocytes, synthesizing and secreting melanin granules), followed by the spinous layer (stratum spinosum), the clear layer (stratum lucidum), the cornified or horny layer (stratum corneum). If there is a problem with the epidermis, it will affect the color and clarity of the skin. The dermis contains collagen fibers, elastic fibers, reticular fibers, and stroma, as well as blood vessels, lymphatic vessels, nerves and skin appendages (hair, sebaceous glands, sweat glands, muscles, etc.). When there is a problem with the dermis, the skin can wrinkle, sag, or develop redness.

The main factors that hinder the cleansing and whitening of the skin are as follows:

Disorders of cell metabolism in the basal layer: formation of stains. Melanin cells that cause pigmentation exist in the basal layer. Under normal conditions, melanin acts like a filter on the skin, protecting the skin and body from damage caused by ultraviolet radiation. If the metabolism of melanin cells is disordered and accumulates in the epidermis, it will cause uneven distribution of pigment, thus forming stains.

Accumulated stratum corneum: rough skin. The stratum corneum is the epidermal cells above the dermis. The accumulation of old keratin disrupts the texture of the skin, which becomes less smooth and loses its clarity.

Abnormal metabolism of the dermis: yellowish skin, sagging, wrinkles. The epidermis is very thin (only 0.1 to 0.3 millimeters thick), and is able to transmit the color of the dermis. The dermis should be pure white, but turns yellow due to glycation and hydroxylation. Skin laxity and wrinkles occur due to abnormalities in collagen fibers, elastic fibers, and reticular fibers.

Increased sebaceous glands secretion: greasy skin. The sebaceous glands secrete too much, resulting in a greasy feeling and enlarged pores.

Poor blood circulation: dull skin. Arteries containing hemoglobin show a healthy reddish color, while veins with less blood oxygen show a greenish color. If there is poor blood flow, the function of internal organs is reduced, and there is a lack of vital *qi*, which results in poor blood mobility. The vein color will appear more obvious, and the complexion will be dull, with dark circles under the eyes.

Using the jade facial *gua sha* scraper to scrape the facial skin stimulates all layers of the skin and subcutaneous tissue, improving the microcirculation of skin cells, promoting skin metabolism, and solving local problems on the face. At the same time, according to the theory of holographic meridians, you can also identify the corresponding meridians and internal organs that cause skin problems, and carry out targeted conditioning to regulate skin color from the inside out in order to obtain clearness and transparency.

Note: Some acupoints discussed in this book are distributed symmetrically on both sides of the body. When conducting facial *gua sha*, except for a few acupoints that require one-sided scraping, all acupoints symmetrical on both sides of the body are to be scraped by default.

Key Points of the Technique

1. Be sure to apply facial *gua sha* cream to the scraping area first.

2. Since the factors that hinder skin whitening may exist in the skin and various layers of tissue under it, the pressing force should penetrate the layers of tissue under the skin, in the muscle, and above the bones. The scraping speed should be slow, with a frequency controlled to 2 to 3 times within one calm breath. Look carefully for positive reactions in dark and lackluster areas. Do not press too hard or too fast.

3. Find the positive reactions in the various tissue under the skin with dullness, and gradually eliminate them by means of pushing and scraping, and kneading and scraping, unblocking the *qi* and blood flow in the meridians, helping to dispel dullness in the skin. It is also necessary to scrape the relevant meridians and holographic corresponding parts of the body to consolidate the effect of facial *gua sha*.

4. A dull complexion is evidence of deficiency syndrome of insufficient *qi* and blood, and even blood stasis. Therefore, scraping must be used to promote blood circulation and remove blood stasis, but it should not be excessive. When the scraped area feels sore, scrape with the tonifying method (light pressure and slow speed).

Dullness on the Forehead

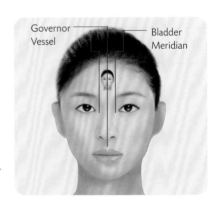

Dullness in the center of the forehead: The center of the forehead is the part where the Governor Vessel and the Bladder Meridian run, and it is also the holographic point of the head, face, neck and throat. Dullness on the forehead is mostly a sign of insufficient kidney *qi*, a *yang qi* deficiency, overuse of the brain, lack of oxygen in the brain, brain fatigue, or neurasthenia.

Facial Beauty *Gua Sha*

1. Apply facial *gua sha* cream, flat-scrape the head area and throat area in the middle of the face (including the Governor Vessel and Bladder Meridian within the head area), to improve the local blood and *qi* circulation.

2. Push and scrape the head area, throat area, the Governor Vessel in the middle of the forehead and the Bladder Meridian area on both sides, focusing on the dull and lusterless parts, scrape 5 times, and look for positive reactions such as gravel, nodules, and pain.

3. Use the kneading and scraping method to scrape the dull area 5 times.

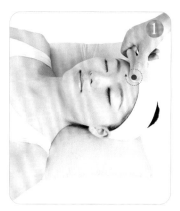
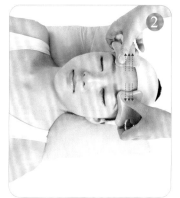
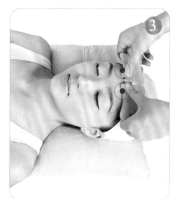

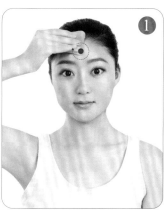
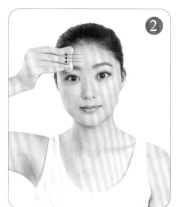
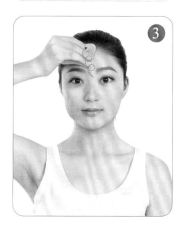

Consolidating *Gua Sha* on the Head and Neck

Scrape the head first: Stimulate the *qi* and blood in the Governor Vessel and the Bladder Meridian, so that the blood of the brain can flow smoothly and the brain can receive rich nutrients.

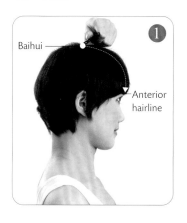
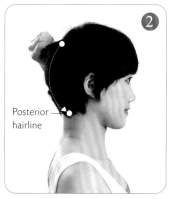
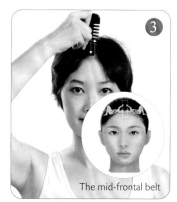

1. Use a scraping comb to scrape the top of the head with the surface-scraping method, from the Baihui acupoint forward to the anterior hairline.

2. Then scrape the back of the head, from the Baihui acupoint backwards to the posterior hairline.

3. Scrape the mid-frontal belt (as shown in the figure on page 67).

Then scrape the neck: Dredge the corresponding area to the head and face on the neck, unbloking *qi* and blood, and improving brain fatigue.

1. Scrape the cervical spine, and use the surface-scraping method on the Governor Vessel in the middle of the back of the neck.

2. Scrape the Bladder Meridian on both sides of the neck with the dual-angle scraping method.

3. Scrape the Fengchi acupoint with the single-angle scraping method, and then use the surface-scraping method downwards from the Fengchi acupoint to the root of neck.

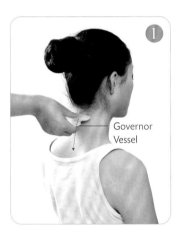
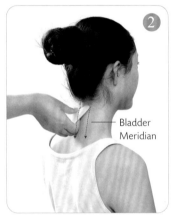
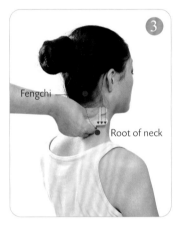

Whole-Body *Gua Sha* and Conditioning

Scrape the lower back through clothes: Tonifies the kidneys and invigorates the *yang qi* of the whole body.

1. Scrape the Governor Vessel on the back from top to bottom through clothes, focusing on the Dazhui acupoint to the Zhiyang and Mingmen acupoints.

2. Enhance the function of the kidneys by scraping from the top downwards the corresponding area of kidneys on the spine using the surface-scraping method.

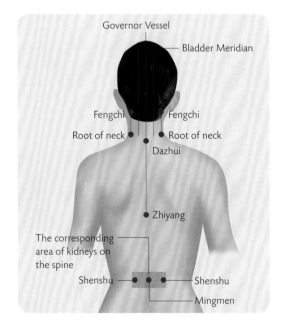

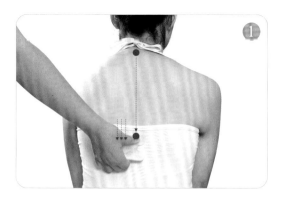

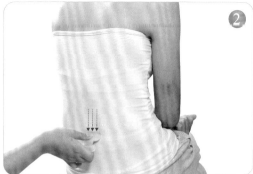

Dullness on both sides of the forehead and near the temples: The two sides of the forehead are the parts where the Gallbladder Meridian and Stomach Meridian run. Dullness in this area is mostly a symptom of liver and gallbladder dysfunction, liver depression and *qi* stagnation, insomnia and excessive dreaming, and irregular menstruation caused by liver blood deficiency or liver depression and *qi* stagnation. Dull and oily foreheads are manifestations of liver stagnation, spleen deficiency, and inner dampness.

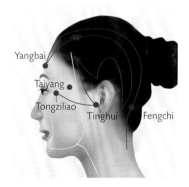

1. Apply facial *gua sha* cream, then scrape the Gallbladder Meridian, Stomach Meridian area, and Taiyang acupoints on both sides of the forehead, focusing on the skin area with dullness, to directly improve local *qi* and blood circulation.

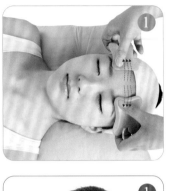 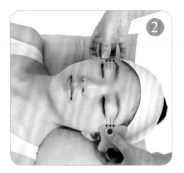 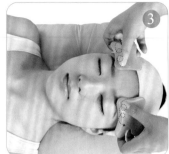

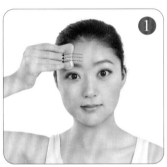 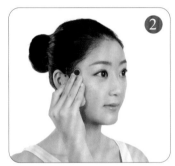 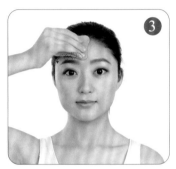

2. Use the pushing and scraping method to focus on the meridians on both sides of the forehead, the Yangbai and Taiyang acupoints, and the positive reaction areas under the dull skin 5 times.

3. Scrape the dull skin area 5 times with the kneading and scraping method.

Consolidating *Gua Sha* on the Head, Neck, and Feet

Scrape the side of the head: Use a scraping comb to scrape the Gallbladder Meridian on the side of the head, from the side of the anterior hairline, draw a question mark along the back of the ear, and scrape down to the posterior hairline. Look for sore points and rough nodules and focus on scraping them. Usually, this area can be scraped every day, for 2 to 3 minutes each time.

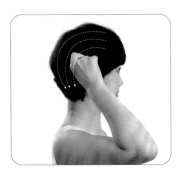 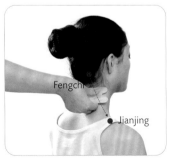 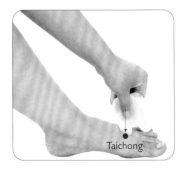

Scrape the neck: Apply scraping oil on the neck and shoulders, then scrape along the side of the neck to the upper shoulders, focus on scraping the Fengchi acupoint with the single-angle scraping method, and scrape the root of neck and Jianjing acupoint with the surface-scraping method. In places where there are positive reaction points such as pain and nodules, perform focused scraping.

Scrape the feet: Use the vertical-pressing and kneading method to press and knead the Taichong acupoint on the feet 5 to 10 times.

Whole-Body *Gua Sha* and Conditioning

1. Scrape the corresponding area of liver and gallbladder on the spine with surface-scraping method, first surface-scrape the Governor Vessel between the 8th and 10th thoracic vertebrae, and then use the dual-angle scraping method to scrape the Jiaji acupoints on both sides of the same horizontal section from top to bottom, then surface-scrape on a 3-cun wide range on both sides of the Governor Vessel from top to bottom.

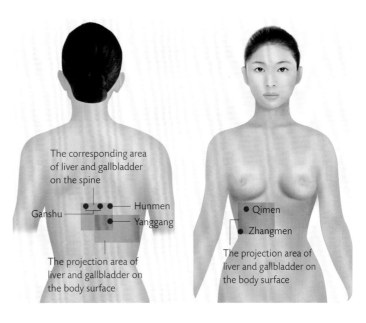

The corresponding area of liver and gallbladder on the spine

Ganshu
Hunmen
Yanggang

The projection area of liver and gallbladder on the body surface

Qimen
Zhangmen

The projection area of liver and gallbladder on the body surface

2. Use the flat-scraping method along the direction of the ribs, and scrape the projection area of liver and gallbladder on the right thoracic region and the right back from the center of the abdomen and back to the right.

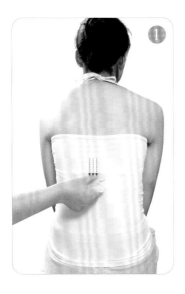

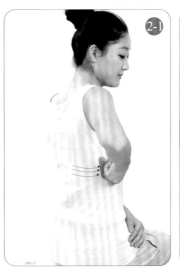

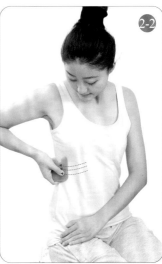

3. Scrape the Ganshu, Hunmen, and Yanggang acupoints from top to bottom for 15 to 20 times with the surface-scraping method.

4. Scrape the Qimen and Zhangmen acupoints from the center of the ribs to both sides for 15 to 20 times with the flat-scraping method.

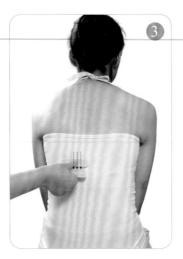
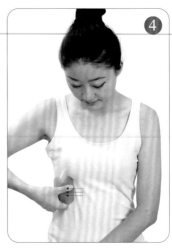

Expert Tips: Tips for Scraping Your Forehead

If the skin on both sides of the forehead is dull and lackluster, this will mostly be due to a stagnation of liver *qi*. Wherever the stagnation of liver *qi* is located, focus on scraping the Liver and Gallbladder Meridians that runs in that part. Look for painful and sensitive points in the area, and focus on scraping them. For the four scraping parts in the "Whole-Body *Gua Sha* and Conditioning" section above, you can only scrape 1, 2 or 3, 4 parts each time. For example, people with dull skin and strong oil secretion often have liver depression, spleen deficiency, and internal dampness. Scrape the Pishu and Weishu acupoints on the back, the Zhongwan acupoint on the abdomen, and the projection area of the spleen on the left side of the abdomen and back.

Dullness around the Eyes

Dullness between the eyebrows: Between the eyebrows is the holographic acupoint area of the lungs. It is also the part where the Governor Vessel and the Bladder Meridian run. Dullness and a lack of luster between the eyebrows is a sign of insufficient lung *qi* and a disorder of *qi* and blood in the lungs. Lung *qi* should be nourished. Dark red between the eyebrows indicates lung heat, which is a sign of chronic inflammation of the throat or elevated blood pressure.

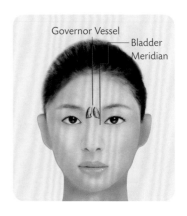

Governor Vessel

Bladder Meridian

Facial Beauty *Gua Sha*

Apply facial *gua sha* cream, then scrape the heart and lung area between the eyebrows with the pushing and scraping method, that is, the forehead Governor Vessel and the

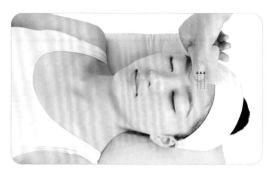
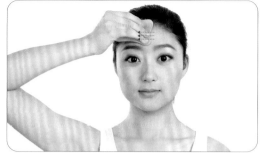

Bladder Meridian area. Focus on scraping the dull and lusterless parts. Scrape 5 times, and look for positive reactions. Use the pushing and scraping method to focus on the positive reaction areas under the meridians, acupoints, and skin with dullness 5 times. Use the flat-pressing and kneading method to scrape the dull area 5 times, until the skin is slightly warm.

Consolidating *Gua Sha* on the Hands and Feet
Scrape the holographic acupoint area for the lungs on the hands and feet.

1. Use a scraper to scrape the lung area of the palm under the little finger with the surface-scraping method, until the skin feels warm.

2. Use the long side of the scraper to scrape the lung area of both feet from top to bottom with the flat-scraping method, until the skin feels warm.

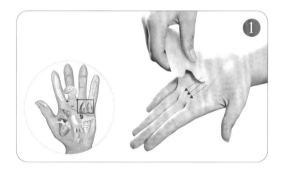
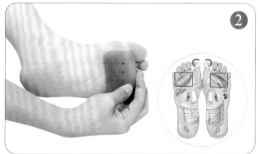

Whole-Body *Gua Sha* and Conditioning

1. Use the surface-scraping method on the corresponding area of heart and lungs on the spine; first scrape the Governor Vessel between the 1st and 9th thoracic vertebrae with the surface-scraping method, and then use the dual-angle

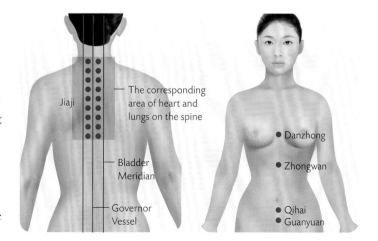

Jiaji

The corresponding area of heart and lungs on the spine

Bladder Meridian

Governor Vessel

Danzhong

Zhongwan

Qihai
Guanyuan

scraping method to scrape the Jiaji acupoints from top to bottom on both sides of the same horizontal section of the Governor Vessel; then use the surface-scraping method on the 3-cun wide area on both sides of the Governor Vessel from top to bottom.

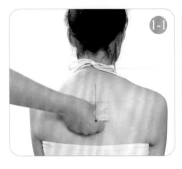
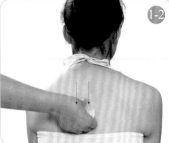
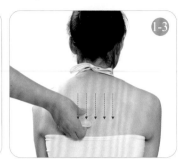

2. Scrape the Taiyuan and Lieque acupoints on the upper limbs from top to bottom with the surface-scraping method.

3. Scrape the Danzhong acupoint on the chest with the single-angle scraping method.

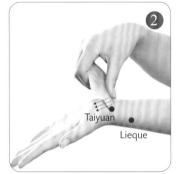
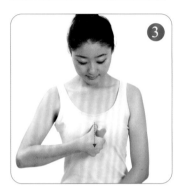

Expert Tip: Scraping for People with a *Qi* Deficiency

The lungs have the physiological function of propelling *qi* and blood through the meridians and transporting them throughout the body, so insufficient lung *qi* will lead to a weakness of vital *qi* throughout the body, making it easy to catch a cold. People with *qi* deficiency should choose a gentle tonifying method for scraping with a low pressing force and slow speed. Each time, the places to be scraped should be minimal and the area should be small. It is most suitable for single acupoint massage and rubbing. Do not pursue producing *sha*, to avoid draining vital *qi*.

Dullness between the eyes: Between the eyes is the holographic point area of the heart, and the area where the Governor Vessel and the Bladder Meridian flow. Pale and lack of luster between the eyes is a sign of heart *qi* deficiency. A slight redness between the eyes is a sign of a flaring up of heart fire; above middle age, redness between the eyebrows and eyes is a sign of increased blood pressure. The appearance of dark red or dark blue

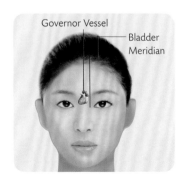

is a sign of deficiency of heart *qi* and blood and blood vessel stagnation, which should be taken seriously. Get plenty of rest, reduce stress, nourish heart *qi*, and carry out physical and mental conditioning.

Facial Beauty *Gua Sha*

1. Apply facial *gua sha* cream, then scrape the heart area between the eyes with the pushing and scraping method (the Governor Vessel area). Focus on scraping the dull and lusterless parts, scraping 5 to 10 times, and looking for any positive reaction.

2. Scrape the dull areas with the flat-pressing and kneading method, and press 5 times until the skin is slightly warm and flushed.

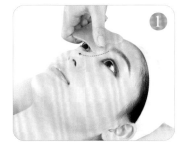
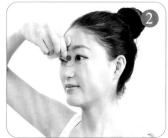

Consolidating *Gua Sha* on the Hands and Feet

Scrape the holographic acupoint area for the heart on the hands and feet to regulate heart function.

1. Use the scraper to scrape the heart area in the thenar with the surface-scraping method, until the skin feels warm.

2. Use the scraper to scrape the heart area on the sole of the left foot from top to bottom using the pushing and scraping method, until the skin feels warm.

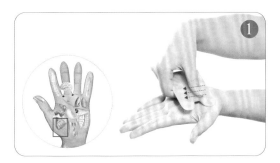
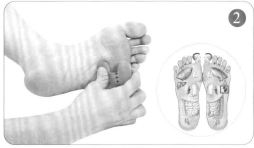

Whole-Body *Gua Sha* and Conditioning

1. Use the surface-scraping method on the corresponding areas of heart and spleen on the spine:
① First scrape the 4th and 8th thoracic vertebrae and the Governor Vessel area

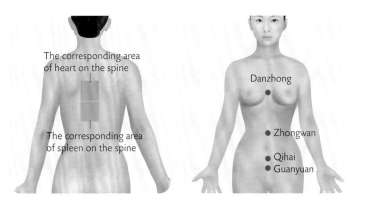

The corresponding area of heart on the spine

The corresponding area of spleen on the spine

Danzhong

Zhongwan

Qihai
Guanyuan

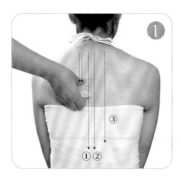
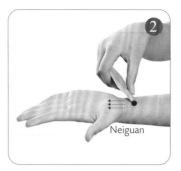
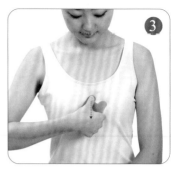

Neiguan

between the 8th to 12th thoracic vertebrae with surface-scraping method. ② Then use the dual-angle scraping method to scrape the Jiaji acupoints from top to bottom on both sides of the same horizontal section of the Governor Vessel. ③ Scrape on a 3-cun wide area on both sides of the Governor Vessel from top to bottom with the surface-scraping method.

2. Use the surface-scraping method on the Neiguan acupoint on the upper limbs from top to bottom.

3. Use the single-angle scraping method to scrape the Danzhong acupoint on the chest from top to bottom.

> **Expert Tip: Conditioning for Heart and Lung *Qi* Deficiency**
>
> The corresponding area of the heart on the face is where *qi* and blood gather, *sha* develop easily here, so the intensity of scraping should be reduced appropriately. If the blood stasis is severe, scrape until a small amount of *sha* occur for better effects. Don't panic—*sha* will disappear quickly within 24 hours.
>
> The holographic acupoints between the eyebrows and the eyes belong to the heart and lung, and the dullness is the external appearance of *qi* and blood deficiency and blood stasis of the heart and lungs. A deficiency of heart *qi* is often accompanied by a deficiency of heart blood, leaving people prone to mental fatigue and forgetfulness, insomnia, and excessive dreaming. When the heart *qi* is deficient, the blood does not have enough power to run, and stagnation in the blood vessels can easily occur, which is the same reason why rivers flow too slowly and are prone to silt. When nourishing heart *qi* and blood deficiency, the heart and spleen should be conditioned together, because the spleen is the source of the production and transformation of *qi* and blood. If the heart *qi* and blood are not nourished from the source, just nourishing the *qi* and blood of the heart alone will leave them without a source, and good results will be hard to achieve. People with weak heart *qi* and blood should keep their spirits up, relax, and not overwork.

Dullness around the eyes: The skin around the eyes is where the Bladder Meridian, Stomach Meridian, Liver Meridian, and Gallbladder Meridian flow. Dull, lackluster skin around the eyes is most likely to appear in the inner corners and lower

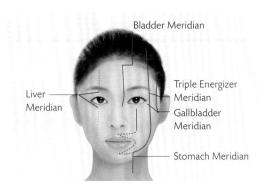

Bladder Meridian

Liver Meridian

Triple Energizer Meridian

Gallbladder Meridian

Stomach Meridian

eyelids, known as dark circles. Dull and black skin around the eyes indicates kidney *qi* deficiency, gastrointestinal dysfunction, irregular menstruation, or lack of sleep and excessive fatigue. Long-term stubborn dark circles indicate overwork, staying up late, or suffering from gynecological diseases, chronic gastrointestinal diseases, chronic liver diseases, and kidney diseases.

Facial Beauty *Gua Sha*

1. For those with dullness in the inner corner of the eyes, apply facial *gua sha* cream, then use the corner of the scraper or the facial *gua sha* scraper for eyes to press and rub the Jingming acupoint with the vertical-pressing and kneading method, move left and right, up and down, and look for positive reactions under the Jingming acupoint. Scrape 5 to 10 times.

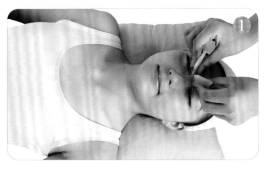
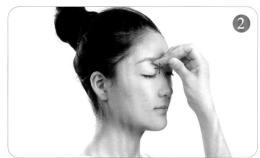
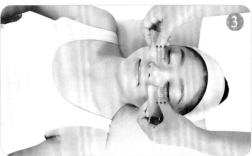
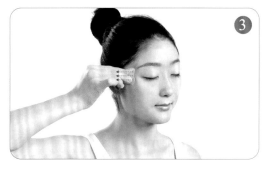

2. Use the pushing and scraping method to slowly push upwards 1 millimeter by 1 millimeter along the Bladder Meridian next to the nose from the Jingming acupoint; push and scrape to the Cuanzhu acupoint, searching for and focusing on scraping the positive reaction areas on the Bladder Meridian and Cuanzhu acupoint 5 to 10 times.

3. If the skin color of the lower eyelid is blue or dull, first scrape the Jingming acupoint according to the above method, and then use the upper part of the long arc of the scraper to scrape from the Jingming acupoint along the lower eye socket to the Tongziliao point at the outer corner of the eye through the Liver Meridian with the

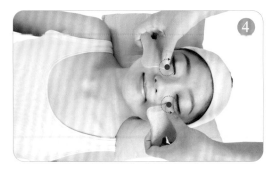

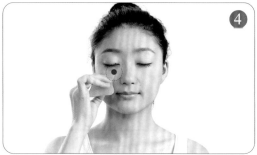

pushing and scraping method. Focus on scraping the Liver Meridian in the middle of the lower eye socket, and find and scrape the positive reaction points 5 to 10 times.

4. Use the flat-pressing and kneading method to slowly press and rub the Chengqi and Sibai acupoints on the lower eyelid 5 times from light to heavy. Look for positive reactions, and then press and rub the positive reaction parts 5 to 10 times.

Consolidating *Gua Sha* on the Head, Neck and Feet

1. Use the sharp-edge scraping method to scrape the second lateral-frontal belt, the third lateral-frontal belt, the Shenting and Meichong acupoints.

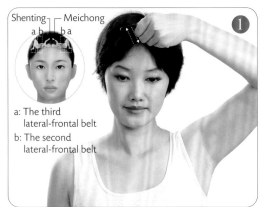

a: The third
lateral-frontal belt
b: The second
lateral-frontal belt

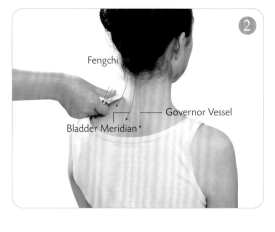

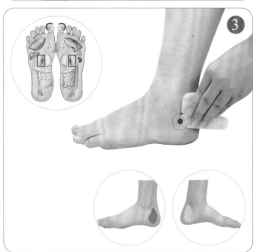

2. Use the surface-scraping and the dual-angle scraping methods to scrape the Governor Vessel on the cervical spine and the Bladder Meridian from top to bottom. Use the single-angle scraping method to scrape the Fengchi acupoint, and then use the surface-scraping method from the Fengchi acupoint down to the root of neck.

3. Scrape the holographic acupoint area of the kidney in the sole, and the holographic acupoint area of the gonad on both inner and outer sides of the heel.

Whole-Body *Gua Sha* and Conditioning

1. Use the surface-scraping method on the Geshu acupoints on the back from top to bottom; also scrape the Ganshu, Danshu and Shenshu acupoints for dull inner corners of the eyes, and scrape the Pishu and Weishu acupoints for dull lower eyelids.

2. Use the surface-scraping and the dual-angle scraping methods to scrape the corresponding area of uterus and ovary on the

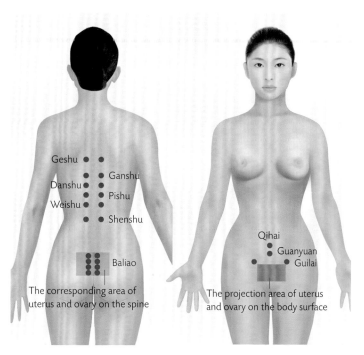

Geshu
Ganshu
Danshu
Pishu
Weishu
Shenshu
Baliao

The corresponding area of uterus and ovary on the spine

Qihai
Guanyuan
Guilai

The projection area of uterus and ovary on the body surface

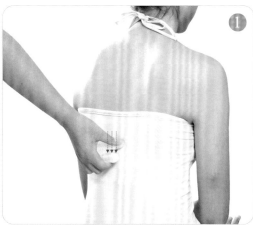

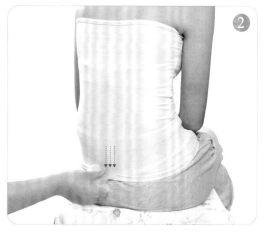

spine from top to bottom, focusing on the Baliao acupoints.

3. Scrape the lower abdomen again to regulate menstruation and invigorate *qi*. Use the surface-scraping method on the projection area of uterus and ovary on the body surface from top to bottom. Then use the surface-scraping method from the Qihai acupoint to the Guanyuan acupoint, and the bilateral Guilai acupoints, from top to bottom.

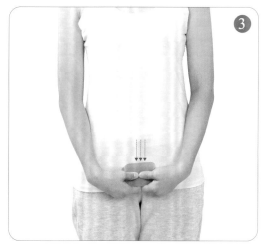

Pale or Dull Nose

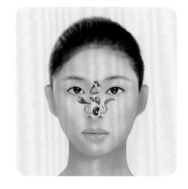

Pale or lackluster nose is the outward sign of a decline in the function of the spleen and stomach and a deficiency of the lungs and spleen. Blackheads on the nose and lack of luster are also signs of spleen and stomach *qi* deficiency; a dull color in the middle of the bridge of the nose is the external sign of liver dysfunction, liver depression and *qi* stagnation. A dark red color on the wings of nose, or on the base of the wings of nose, is a sign of stomach *qi* dysfunction, with the depression transforming into heat. If the wings of nose and the base of the wings of nose are dark and lack luster, this indicates stomach *qi* deficiency and stomach deficiency-cold. A dark blue nose tip indicates spleen deficiency-cold, cold pain in the abdomen, and lack of warmth in the hands and feet.

Facial Beauty *Gua Sha*

1. Apply facial *gua sha* cream, then use the long arc of the scraper to push and scrape the center of the nose bridge from the root of nose to the tip. Identify and scrape the positive reaction points 5 to 10 times.

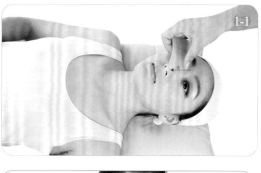
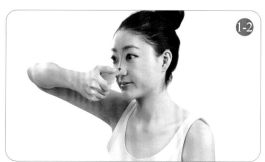
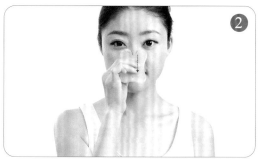
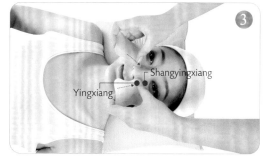

2. Scrape the gallbladder area, pancreas area, stomach area, and nasal groove on the side of the nose with the pushing and scraping method. Find and scrape the positive reaction points 5 to 10 times.

3. Use the pushing and scraping method to scrape the Shangyingxiang and Yingxiang acupoints. Find and press and knead the positive reaction points.

Consolidating *Gua Sha* on the Head, Hands, and Feet

1. Use the sharp-edge scraping method to scrape the second lateral-frontal belt on both sides of the head.

2. Use the surface-scraping method on the thenar of the palm.

3. Use the surface-scraping method on the stomach area in the sole and the liver and gallbladder areas of the right foot.

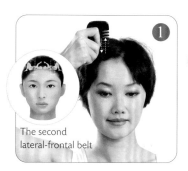
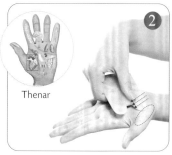
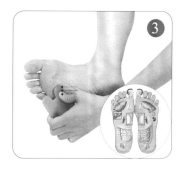

Whole-Body *Gua Sha* and Conditioning

1. Use the surface-scraping method on the corresponding areas of liver, gallbladder, spleen, pancreas on the spine. ① Use the surface-scraping method on the Governor Vessel between the 8th and 12th thoracic vertebrae first. ② Use the dual-angle scraping method to scrape the Jiaji acupoints from top to bottom on both sides at the same horizontal section of the Governor Vessel. ③ Use the surface-scraping method on the 3-cun wide area on both sides of the Governor Vessel from top to bottom. Focus on scraping the Yishu, Ganshu, Danshu, Pishu, and Weishu acupoints on the back. For people with pale and lacklusters noses, just scrape the key points.

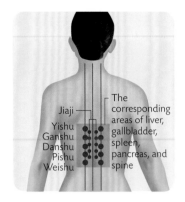

2. Use the surface-scraping method on the Zusanli and Yinlingquan acupoints on the lower limbs from top to bottom, and use the vertical-pressing and kneading method to scrape the Taichong acupoints on the feet.

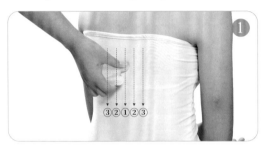

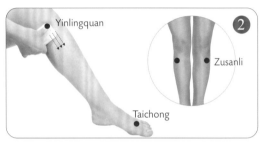

Expert Tips: The Role of Innate and Acquired Foundations

The kidneys are innate foundation, while the spleen and stomach are acquired foundation. This refers to the foundation of life. According to traditional Chinese medicine, the innate part related to heredity is managed by the kidneys, and the acquired part related to diet is managed by the spleen and stomach.

Here we must first clarify a concept. The heart, liver, spleen, lungs, and kidneys in Western medicine refer to real tangible organs, while in TCM they are a functional system. For example, the spleen in Western medicine refers simply to the organ called the spleen, but in TCM it is equivalent to an energy base of the human body. It transports the refined substances in the food to all parts of the body. Essence is food nutrition which has gone through processing by the spleen, which is equivalent to decomposing protein into amino acids, because it becomes very small, so TCM calls it the essence of food and drink. This process of turning food into very small and refined substances is the transportation and transformation function of the spleen. TCM summarizes the process of decomposing food as "transformation," and the process of absorbing refined substances by the human body as "transportation," which is equivalent to the two complete processes of digestion and absorption we are talking about now.

Red, Dull, or Pale Cheek Areas

Redness and dullness in the center of the cheek areas suggest an accumulation of heat in the small intestine or *qi* and blood stasis in the Heart Meridian, slow blood flow, depression or irritability. Pallor and a lack of luster on the cheek areas suggests a deficiency of heart *qi* and blood.

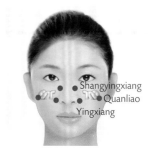

Shangyingxiang
Quanliao
Yingxiang

Facial Beauty *Gua Sha*

1. Scrape the small intestine area and Shangyingxiang acupoint on the face with the pushing and scraping method.

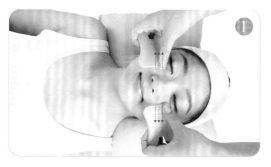
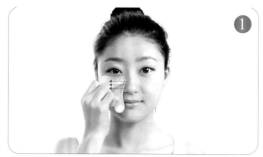
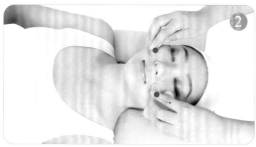
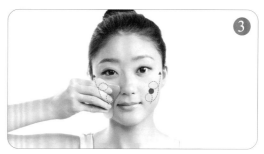

    2. Use the long arc edge of the scraper to push the Quanliao acupoint from bottom to top. Find and scrape the positive reaction points 5 to 10 times.

    3. Press and knead the small intestine area and the Yingxiang acupoint with the flat-pressing and kneading method, and scrape the Quanliao acupoint and the red and dull parts of the two cheek areas with the kneading and scraping method.

Consolidating *Gua Sha* on the Head, Hands, and Feet

1. Use the sharp-edge scraping method to scrape the first lateral-frontal belt and the second lateral-frontal belt on both sides of the head.

    2. Use the surface-scraping method on the thenar of the palm, the heart area and the small intestine area of the left foot.

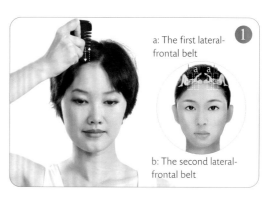

a: The first lateral-frontal belt

b: The second lateral-frontal belt

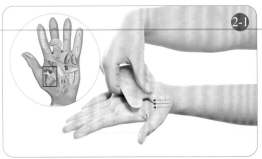
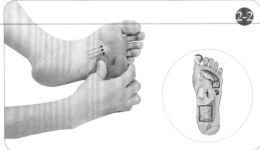

Whole-Body *Gua Sha* and Conditioning

1. Scrape the corresponding area of heart on the spine with the surface-scraping method. First use the surface-scraping method to focus scraping on the Governor Vessel between the 4th to 8th thoracic vertebrae, and then use

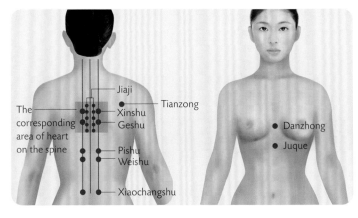

the dual-angle scraping method to scrape the Jiaji acupoints from top to bottom on both sides of the same horizontal section with the Governor Vessel. Then use the surface scraping method to scrape the 3-cun wide range on both sides of the Governor Vessel from top to bottom. Scrape the Xinshu, Geshu, Xiaochangshu, and Tianzong acupoints. For people with pale and lackluster cheekbones, just scrape the key points.

2. Use the single-angle scraping method to scrape the Danzhong and Juque

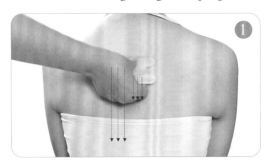
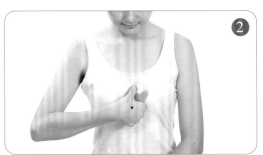
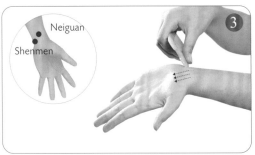
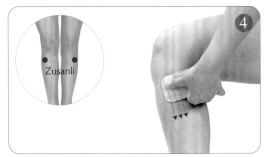

acupoints from top to bottom.

3. Scrape the Shenmen and Neiguan acupoints with the surface-scraping method from top to bottom, or press and knead the points with the flat-pressing and kneading method.

4. People with pale and lackluster cheekbones are suffering from a deficiency of heart *qi*. Scrape with the tonifying method, removing the Geshu acupoint, and adding stimulation to the Pishu, Weishu, and Zusanli acupoints on the basis of the previous steps.

Expert Tips: *Gua Sha* to Promote Blood Circulation and Remove Blood Stasis

If both cheekbones are red, dull and lackluster, or if chloasma appears, blood stasis is the most common cause. The reasons for the formation of blood stasis are very complex. Blood flows in the blood vessels, much like rivers in nature, flowing endlessly. The difference is that the "rivers" in the human body are completely closed, and power is needed to return the blood in the veins to the arteries—more like the circulating water in an ecological fish tank. In the human body, this power is the heart *qi*, which drives the blood circulation back and forth. If the heart *qi* is deficient and power is insufficient, the flow rate will slow down and the volume will decrease. As well as being driven by the heart *qi*, the blood flow in the blood vessels also depends on liver *qi* for conveyance and dispersion. Liver *qi* ensures the correct flow of *qi* and blood. Therefore, emotional depression or excessive mental stress will affect the liver's conveyance and dispersion abilities, as well as the smooth flow of the blood vessels. This is like the water-circulating pipe in a fish tank being blocked. In nature, if the temperature is too low, water will freeze; if the temperature is too high, it will evaporate into steam. If the pressure in a closed container is too high, it will also affect the flow of water, and may even cause the container to burst. The blood in the blood vessels will also be affected by changes in body temperature, which may decelerate the flow rate or cause blood vessel stasis.

The degree of blood vessel stasis will be reflected on the face. Slight blood vessel stasis is manifested by unclear skin color. Dull skin and chloasma are more serious external manifestations of *qi* and blood stasis in the body. The scraper can clear blood stasis and promote blood circulation, with direct and rapid effect.

Dullness of the Upper Part of the Lips

Dullness and lack of luster of the skin under the nose and above the lips can be caused by a variety of reasons: First, it is a sign of deficiency-cold in the large intestine or bladder, which can lead to constipation or weak urination; second, it is a sign of uterine and ovarian dysfunction and endocrine disorders, which can be characterized by coldness and pain in the lower abdomen, and irregular menstruation.

If the color of the philtrum is dull and the grooves are dark, it is a sign of a lack of *yang qi*; bulging groove is mostly seen in men with prostate hypertrophy, and in women with pregnancy or uterine disorders. If the skin around the mouth is blue and dull, it suggests that the spleen and stomach and the lower *jiao* are deficiency-cold. In addition to the above symptoms, there may also be stomach cold, stomach pain, and a preference for hot beverages.

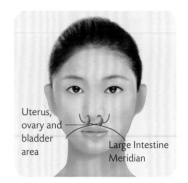

Facial Beauty *Gua Sha*

Methods of scraping for others: Apply facial *gua sha* cream, and scrape the Renzhong acupoint, the uterus area, the Kouheliao acupoint, the ovary area, the bladder area, the Dicang acupoint, and the Yingxiang acupoint with the pushing and scraping method. Look for and scrape the positive reaction areas for 5 to 10 times each.

Self-scraping method: Use the flat-pressing and kneading method to scrape the Renzhong acupoint, uterus area, the ovary area, the bladder area, the Heliao acupoint, Dicang acupoint, and Yingxiang acupoint 5 times each.

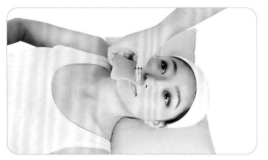

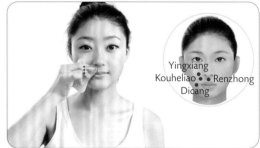

Consolidating *Gua Sha* on the Head, Hands, and Feet

1. Use the sharp-edge scraping method to scrape the mid-frontal belt and the third lateral-frontal belt on both sides.

2. Use the surface-scraping method on the hypothenar and the large intestine area in the sole, and use the push-scraping method to scrape the gonad area on both sides of the heel and in the sole.

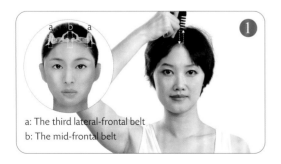

a: The third lateral-frontal belt
b: The mid-frontal belt

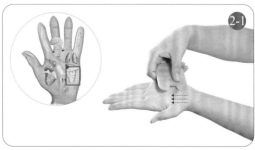

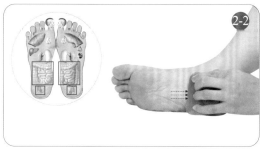

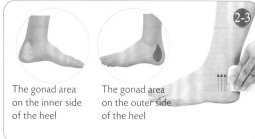

The gonad area on the inner side of the heel

The gonad area on the outer side of the heel

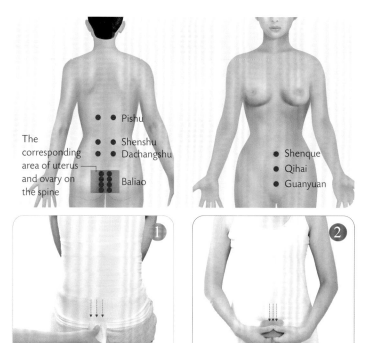

The corresponding area of uterus and ovary on the spine

Pishu

Shenshu
Dachangshu

Baliao

Shenque
Qihai
Guanyuan

Whole-Body *Gua Sha* and Conditioning

1. Scrape the corresponding area of uterus and ovary on the spine. First use the surface-scraping method on the Governor Vessel in the middle of the 2nd and 4th sacral vertebrae, then use the dual-angle scraping method to scrape the Baliao points on both sides at the same time. Use the surface-scraping method to scrape a 3-cun wide range on both sides of the sacrum. Focus on scraping the Pishu, Shenshu, Dachangshu, and Baliao acupoints on both sides.

2. Scrape the Qihai and Guanyuan acupoints from top to bottom for 5 to 10 strokes with the surface-scraping method.

3. Use the surface-scraping method on the Quchi acupoint on the upper limbs, and the Zusanli and Sanyinjiao acupoints on the lower limbs from top to bottom.

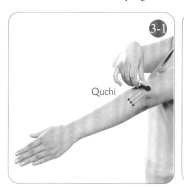

Quchi

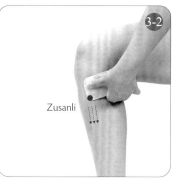

Zusanli

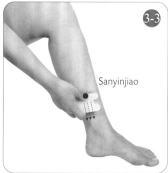

Sanyinjiao

The lips are the window for observing the strength of the spleen function. The skin on the upper part of the lips is the part where the Large Intestine Meridian flows, and it is also the part corresponding to the reproductive organs of the ovaries and uterus, the prostate, and the urinary bladder. These organs belong to the lower *jiao* in TCM. TCM divides the human body into upper, middle and lower *jiao*. The heart and lungs above the diaphragm belong to the upper *jiao*; the liver, gallbladder, spleen, and stomach in the upper abdomen below the diaphragm belong to the middle *jiao*; and the kidneys, bladder, reproductive organs, large intestine, and small intestine in the lower abdomen belong to the lower *jiao*.

When the lower *jiao* is damp and hot, the urine will be yellowish, the stool will be sticky and unclear, and the upper lip area will show acne or oil secretion. When the lower *jiao* has deficiency-cold, there will often be cold and painful abdominal discomfort, a preference for warmth and pressure in the lower abdomen, and irregular menstruation. The upper lip area will show changes such as dullness and lack of luster or development of spots and blemishes. People with a healthy spleen and stomach and normal function of the lower *jiao* organs will have moist upper lip skin.

Dullness of the Lower Jaw

Dullness and lack of luster in the jaw area are signs of kidney *qi* deficiency, cold in the uterus, endocrine disorders, lumbago, and menstrual disorders.

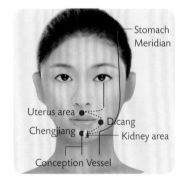

Facial Beauty *Gua Sha*
1. Apply facial *gua sha* cream, and scrape the Chengjiang acupoint and uterus area with the pushing and scraping method, then push and scrape from the Chengjiang acupoint to the Dicang acupoint. Find and focus on the positive reaction points, scraping 5 to 10 times.

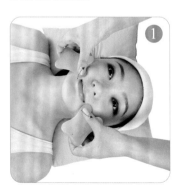
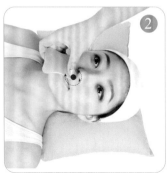
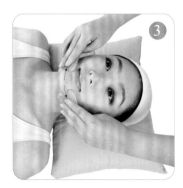

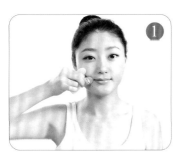 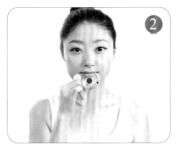 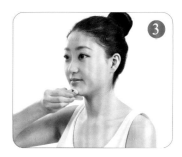

2. Scrape the Chengjiang acupoint, the uterus area of the upper lip, and the kidney area of the lower jaw with the flat-pressing and kneading method.

3. Use the groove at the corner of the scraper to scrape the Conception Vessel and the Stomach Meridian areas on the lower jaw with the pushing and scraping method. Find and focus on the positive reaction points for 5 to 10 times.

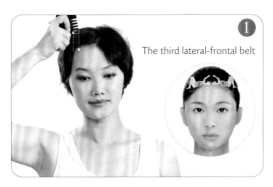

The third lateral-frontal belt

Consolidating *Gua Sha* on the Head, Hands, and Feet

1. Use the sharp-edge scraping method to scrape the third lateral-frontal belt on both sides of the head.

2. Use the surface-scraping method on the hypothenar, and use the pushing and scraping method to scrape the gonad area in the sole and on both sides of the heel.

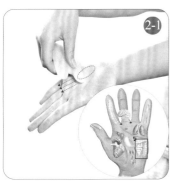 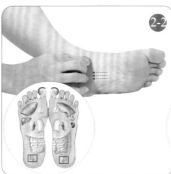 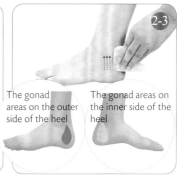

The gonad areas on the outer side of the heel

The gonad areas on the inner side of the heel

Whole-Body *Gua Sha* and Conditioning

1. Use the surface-scraping method and the dual-angle scraping method to scrape the corresponding area of uterus and ovary on spine at the lumbosacral region from top to bottom. ① Use the surface-scraping method on the Governor Vessel between the 2nd and 4th sacral vertebra first. ② Use the dual-angle scraping method on the Bladder Meridian on both sides of the same horizontal section of the Governor Vessel from top to bottom. ③ Use the surface-scraping method on the 3-cun wide area on both sides of the sacrum from top to bottom. Focus on the Shenshu and Baliao acupoints on both sides.

2. Use the surface-scraping method to scrape the Qihai and Guanyuan acupoints

through clothing from top to bottom until the local area feels hot.

3. Use the surface-scraping method on the Sanyinjiao and Yongquan acupoints of the lower limbs from top to bottom.

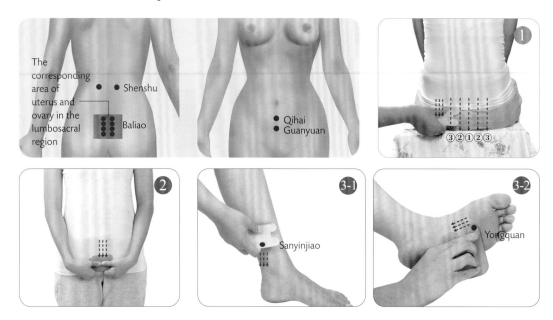

Expert Tip: Enough Kidney Essence Means Plump, Moist Mouth and Lips

The skin of the lower lip is the circulation area of the Stomach Meridian, and the Chengjiang acupoint area below the lower lip corresponds to the kidneys and reflects the health of the uterus. The Renzhong acupoint area on the upper lip corresponds to the uterus, while the Chengjiang acupoint is the counterpart of the uterus. This is because the Renzhong acupoint is part of the Governor Vessel and the Chengjiang acupoint is part of the Conception Vessel, both of which originate in the uterus in women and the prostate in men. The two points—one *yang* and one *yin*—reflect the strength and weakness of the *yin* and *yang* of the reproductive organs. If *yin* and *yang* are balanced and *qi* and blood are harmonized, the jaw will be rounded, the lips red and full, and the skin moist.

Women have different physiological processes from men, and these processes are closely related to the uterus. In TCM theory, the function of the ovaries is attributed to the uterus. It is therefore easy to understand why our appearance is so closely related to the uterus. It is the estrogen secreted by the ovaries that maintains a woman's graceful body and smooth, radiant skin. Once the ovaries atrophy and estrogen decreases, a woman's skin will lose its moist, plump beauty and become dry and yellowish, or even gloomy and dull.

When there is a problem here, it is not only necessary to scrape the local area, but also to condition the corresponding areas of the uterus and ovaries on the back and abdomen for positive and long-lasting results.

Dullness on the Lateral Sides of the Lower Jaw

Dullness on the lateral sides of the lower jaw (both cheeks) is a symptom of insufficient *qi* and blood in the lower limbs, poor blood circulation, soreness and coldness in the lower limbs, insufficient *yang qi* in the stomach, and deficiency-cold in the Stomach Meridian.

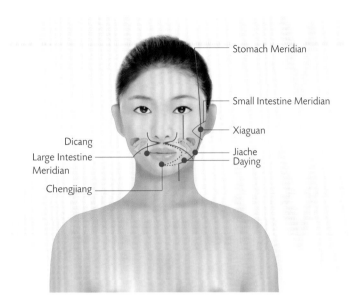

Stomach Meridian

Small Intestine Meridian

Xiaguan

Dicang

Large Intestine Meridian

Jiache
Daying

Chengjiang

Facial Beauty *Gua Sha*

1. Apply facial *gua sha* cream. First use the pushing and scraping method to scrape the Dicang, Daying, and Chengjiang acupoints to the Jiache and Xiaguan acupoints along the Stomach Meridian. Find and focus on the positive reaction points. Scrape 5 to 10 times each.

2. Use the pushing and scraping method to scrape the lower limb area. Find and focus on the positive reaction points. Scrape 5 to 10 times each.

3. Use the groove at the corner of the scraper to scrape the Large Intestine Meridian, Stomach Meridian, and Small Intestine Meridian areas of the lower jaw 5 times each with the pushing and scraping method.

4. Scrape the lower limb area with the kneading and scraping method.

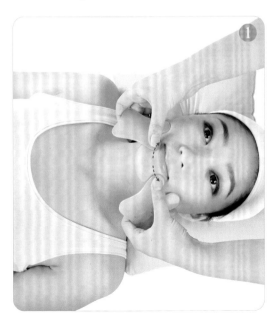

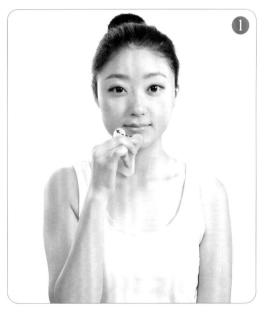

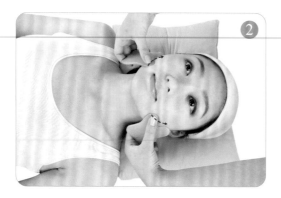

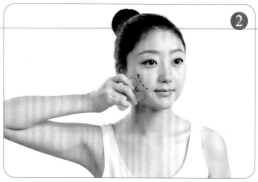

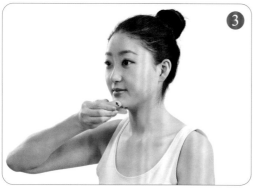

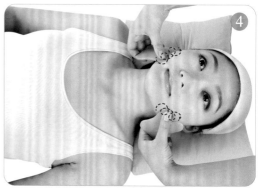

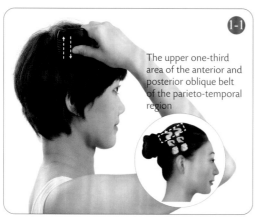

The upper one-third area of the anterior and posterior oblique belt of the parieto-temporal region

Consolidating *Gua Sha* on the Head and Hands

1. Use the sharp-edge scraping method to scrape the third lateral-frontal belt on both sides of the head, as well as the upper one third area of the anterior and posterior oblique belt of the parieto-temporal region.

    2. Scrape each finger with the groove of the scraper.

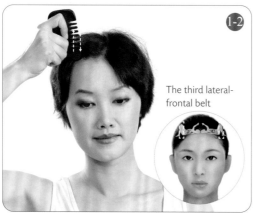

The third lateral-frontal belt

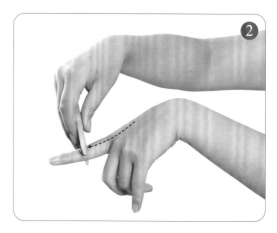

Whole-Body *Gua Sha* and Conditioning

1. Use the surface-scraping method on the Dazhu, Pishu, Weishu, and Shenshu acupoints on both sides of the back from top to bottom.

    2. Use the surface-scraping method on the Yanglingquan, Zusanli, Juegu, and Yongquan acupoints on the lower limbs from top to bottom.

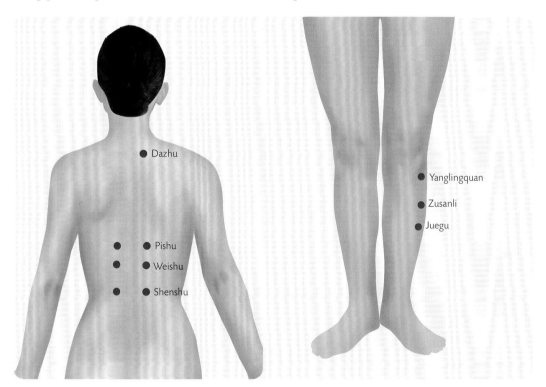

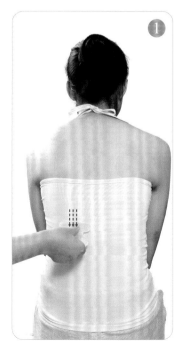

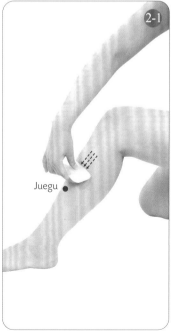

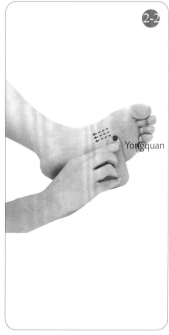

Expert Tip: A Healthy Spleen and Stomach Lead to a Good Complexion

The outer lower jaw is the part where the Stomach Meridian runs on the face, and can reflect the fluctuations of *qi* and blood in the Stomach Meridian. The Stomach Meridian is the longest meridian line on the face, and is most closely related to physical appearance. If you observe carefully at the dinner table, you can see that people who eat and drink enough have rich stomach *qi*, and their complexions are naturally ruddy and shiny. Some people go on a diet to lose weight, and their complexion immediately becomes dull.

From the holographic distribution of the face, this area corresponds to the lower limbs, so if the Stomach Meridian is deficient in *qi* and blood, the muscles are malnourished, and the lower limbs will be sore and weak. Spleen-stomach *qi* deficiency can also lead to lower *jiao* deficiency-cold, soreness, weakness of the waist and knees, and cold lower limbs. Strengthening the spleen and nourishing the stomach is not only related to beauty, but also to health. The simplest and most practical way to tonify the spleen and stomach is to eat the right food in the right amount—neither too much (which will tire the organs) nor too little to starve the organs. This is the best way to tonify your spleen and stomach and beautify your appearance.

Diet Therapy and Skin Care

• People with darker or yellower complexions should eat food rich in vitamin C. Regular consumption of peas and carrots can inhibit the formation of pigments.

• People with rough skin and thick stratum corneum should eat more food with high vitamin A and vitamin B2 content. Shiitake mushrooms, lily bulbs, and coix seeds help improve skin quality.

• People with dry skin should eat more food with slightly higher fat content and rich vitamin E. Drink honey water frequently to nourish the skin and make it soft, white, and smooth.

• People with oily skin should choose food rich in sugar and vitamin C, such as rapeseed, tomato, Chinese cabbage, leek, shepherd's purse, hawthorn berries, citrus, fresh dates, kiwi, and lemons.

• Eat wolfberry, black sesame, and cherry frequently to nourish the skin and delay skin aging.

Food Therapy Recipes

• Take an appropriate amount of tomato, cucumber, lemon, and fresh rose petals. Wash and squeeze them together to extract the juice, then add honey and drink at any time. Drinking this juice frequently can promote skin metabolism, eliminate pigmentation, and make the skin soft, clear, and delicate.

• Wash 10 grams of ginseng. Soak 25 grams of white fungus until it swells and wash well. Cook one egg and peel off the skin. Put the three ingredients into water and cook for two hours on low heat. Add honey to taste after cooling. Regular consumption can make complexion soft, clear, and ruddy.

• Take 20 grams of black fungus, 30 grams of red dates, and 100 grams of rice. Soak the black fungus in clean water until it swells and wash it. Wash the red dates and remove the pits. Wash the rice, and cook the three ingredients together to make porridge. Eat it in the morning and evening to promote blood circulation, purify the skin, and tonify the *qi* and blood.

• Take 50 grams each of wolfberry and longan flesh, and an appropriate amount of honey. Wash the wolfberry and longan flesh. Put them in a pot, add water, and boil slowly over a low heat. Cook until the flesh is desugared, then turn off the heat. After cooling, mix with honey, and eat at any time to soothe the nerves, nourish the blood, and moisturize the skin.

CHAPTER FIVE
Smoothing Wrinkles and Firming the Skin

Wrinkles are the manifestation of skin aging. As we age, the skin's ability to produce collagen and elastic fibers decreases, and the content will gradually decrease, resulting in thinning of the dermis and weakening of density and elasticity, making the skin appear wrinkled and sagging.

From the point of view of traditional Chinese medicine, wrinkles are caused by insufficient *qi* and blood, and a lack of nutrition. However, the first wrinkles that appear on the face are not in the same place for everyone. Even at the same age, the number and depth of wrinkles are obviously different for each person. This is because epidermal wrinkles are the external manifestation of the aging of the internal organs and *qi* and blood deficiency. The skin on different parts of the face is governed by different meridians and visceral organs. By observing where wrinkles appear, it is possible to ascertain which of the viscera begin to age first. By observing the changes in the depth and quantity of wrinkles, we can understand the aging process of the viscera and meridians.

Note: Some acupoints involved in this book are distributed symmetrically on both sides of the body. When conducting facial *gua sha*, except for a few acupoints that require one-sided scraping, the rest are all symmetrical acupoints on both sides of the body by default.

Key Points of the Technique

1. Be sure to apply facial *gua sha* cream on the treatment area first.

2. To lighten fine wrinkles, the pressure should be relatively light, penetrating the soft tissue under the skin and above the muscles. To improve loose skin or deep and obvious wrinkles, the pressure should be slightly greater, penetrating deep into the muscles.

3. The speed of scraping should be slow, controlled to scraping 2 to 3 times within one calm breath. Do not press too hard or scrape too fast. The angle of the wrinkle-reducing *gua sha* method should be small. It is best to press the scraper flat on the wrinkles, and perform flat-scraping method or flat-pressing and kneading method slowly.

4. Determine the direction of scraping according to the shape of the wrinkles: Horizontal wrinkles should be scraped upwards, longitudinal wrinkles should be scraped stretching out horizontally, oblique nasolabial folds should be scraped outwards and upwards, and radial crow's feet should be applied with flat-pressing and kneading method and flat-scraping method outward and upward.

5. Wrinkles are a manifestation of *qi* and blood deficiency. Therefore, the meridians and visceral organs corresponding to wrinkles should be regulated and tonified. All parts of the body should be scraped with the tonifying method, and the time for each session should not be too long.

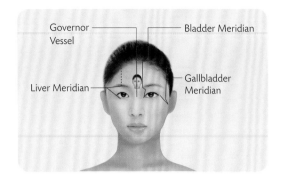

Governor Vessel — Bladder Meridian
Liver Meridian — Gallbladder Meridian

Forehead Wrinkles

Wrinkles in the middle of the forehead are a sign of *qi* and blood deficiency in the brain, fatigue, and neurasthenia. Wrinkles on both sides of the forehead and at the Taiyang acupoints are a sign of *qi* and blood deficiency and weakened functions of liver and gallbladder.

Facial Beauty *Gua Sha*

1. Apply facial *gua sha* cream; first, press and knead the wrinkled parts in the middle of the forehead and the throat area 5 times each with the flat-pressing and kneading method, and then use the flat-scraping method to scrape 5 to 10 times on the horizontal wrinkles in the middle of the forehead from bottom to top. For longitudinal wrinkles, scrape 5 to 10 times horizontally until the skin is slightly warm.

2. First, press and knead the wrinkles of the Gallbladder Meridian on both sides of the forehead with the flat-pressing and kneading method 5 times, and use the pushing and scraping method to scrape the Yangbai point from the inside to the outside. Then, use the flat-scraping method to scrape the wrinkles from bottom to top 5 to 10 times

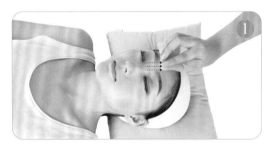

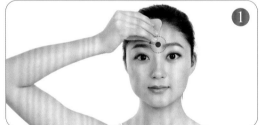

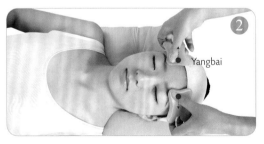

Yangbai

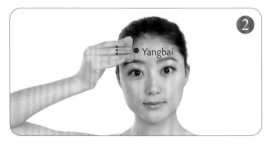

Yangbai

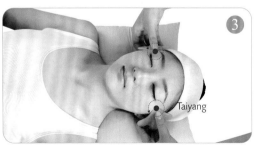

Taiyang

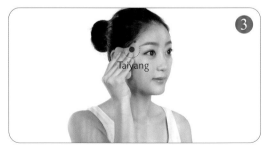

Taiyang

until the skin is slightly warm.

3. Press and knead the wrinkles on the Taiyang acupoints 5 times with the flat-pressing and kneading method, and then use the flat-scraping method to scrape 5 to 10 times from the inside to the outside until the skin is slightly warm.

Consolidating *Gua Sha* on the Head, Hands and Feet

1. For wrinkles in the middle of the forehead, first use the single-angle scraping method to scrape the Shenting and Meichong points on the forehead, then use the surface-scraping method to scrape from the Baihui point on the top of the head to the front hairline, and then scrape back from the Baihui acupoint to the back of the head. Focus on the Baihui acupoint. If wrinkles appear on both sides of the forehead, use the single-angle scraping method to scrape the Toulinqi and Benshen acupoints on the front of the head, then place the scraper vertically on the edge of the hairline on the upper part of the ear, and scrape the sides of the head from front to back around the ear.

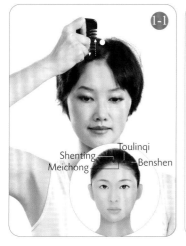
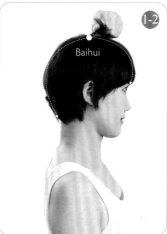
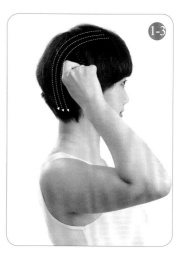

2. Use one side of the scraper to scrape the lung area under the little finger on the palm with the surface-scraping method until the skin in this area feels warm.

3. Use one side of the scraper to scrape the lung area of both feet with the surface-scraping method until the skin in this area feels warm.

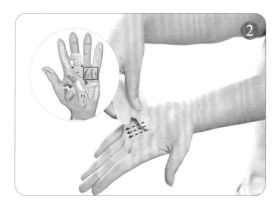
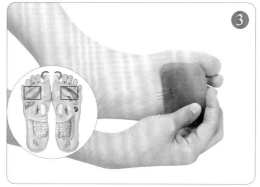

Whole-Body *Gua Sha* and Conditioning

1. Apply *gua sha* oil on the cervical spine region. If there are wrinkles in the middle of the forehead, first scrape the Governor Vessel in the middle of the cervical spine. Use the surface-scraping method to scrape from the Yamen acupoint to the Dazhui acupoint, and then use the dual-angle scraping method to simultaneously scrape from the Tianzhu acupoint to the Dazhu acupoint on both sides. If there are wrinkles on both sides of the forehead, first use the single-angle scraping method to scrape the Fengchi acupoint from top to bottom, and then continue downward using the surface-scraping method to scrape along the Gallbladder Meridian on the neck.

2. Scrape the Ganshu, Danshu, and Shenshu acupoints on the back from top to bottom with the surface-scraping method.

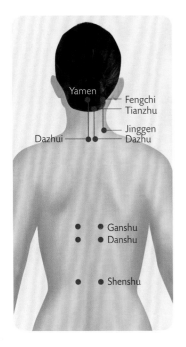
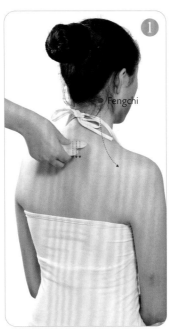
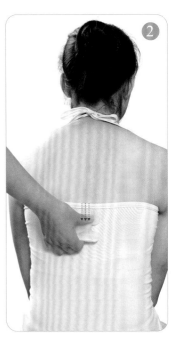

3. Press and knead the Taichong and Xiaxi acupoints on the foot with the vertical pressing and kneading method, and the Yongquan acupoint in the sole with the flat-pressing and kneading method.

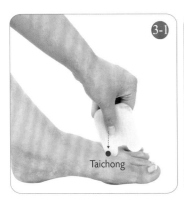
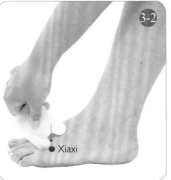
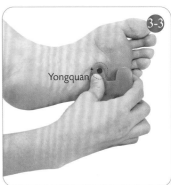

The Gallbladder Meridian runs across the two sides of the forehead. To prevent and improve wrinkles in this area, one should avoid overthinking. One should also pay attention to maintaining the liver and gallbladder to avoid liver blood deficiency caused by an excessive burden on the liver and gallbladder, or malnutrition. The center of the forehead is where the Governor Vessel and Bladder Meridian run. To prevent and improve wrinkles in the center of the forehead, *qi* should be strengthened and the kidneys should be nourished, excessive use of the brain and depletion of *yang qi* should be avoided.

Neck muscle strain, and aging and thinning of the cervical intervertebral disc can also be reflected in the face as early forehead wrinkles. Therefore, good cervical spine health can prevent degenerative cervical changes and early forehead wrinkles.

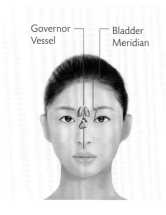

Governor Vessel — Bladder Meridian

Wrinkles between the Eyebrows and Eyes

Between the eyebrows and eyes is the holographic acupoint area of the heart and lungs. It is also the circulation course of the Governor Vessel and the Bladder Meridian. Wrinkles between the eyebrows are a sign of deficiencies in lung *qi* and blood. Wrinkles between the eyes are a sign of deficiency of both *qi* and blood of heart. Avoid mental fatigue and depleting *qi*, and take plenty of rest. Nourishing the *qi* of the heart and lungs is the best way to prevent and relieve wrinkles.

Facial Beauty *Gua Sha*

1. Apply facial *gua sha* cream. Rub the throat area in the middle and lower part of the forehead, the lung area and the heart area between the two eyebrows and eyes with the flat-pressing and kneading method, and scrape each part 5 to 10 times.

2. Use the flat-scraping method to scrape the heart area and lung area slowly at the base of the nose from bottom to top, until the skin is slightly hot and flushed.

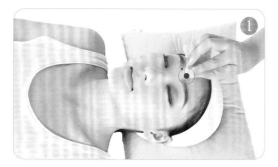

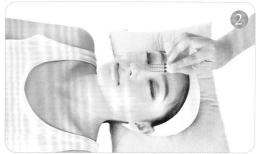

Consolidating *Gua Sha* on the Hands and Feet

1. Use one side of the scraper to scrape the heart area on the thenar and the lung area under the little finger with the surface-scraping method, until the skin in this area feels warm.

2. Use the long side of the scraper to scrape the lung area of both feet and the heart area on the left sole from top to bottom using the flat-scraping method until the skin feels warm.

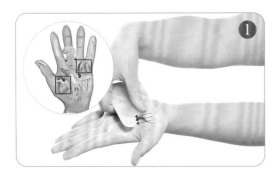
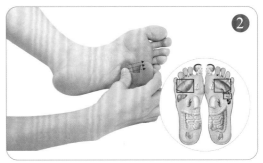

Whole-Body *Gua Sha* and Conditioning

1. Scrape the Governor Vessel, and the Feishu, Xinshu, and Shenshu acupoints on the back with the surface-scraping method from top to bottom with the tonifying method.

2. Scrape the Danzhong acupoint from top to bottom with the single-angle scraping method.

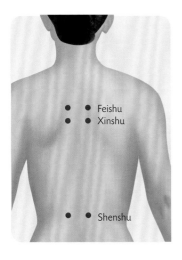
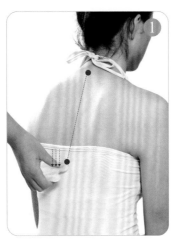
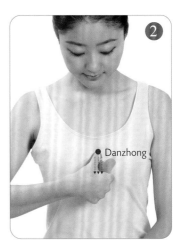

3. Massage the Neiguan acupoint with the flat-pressing and kneading method.

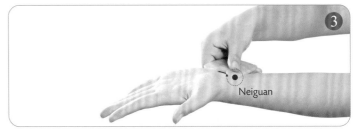

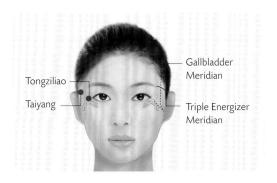

Tongziliao

Taiyang

Gallbladder Meridian

Triple Energizer Meridian

Wrinkles around the Eyes

Crow's feet at the corners of the eyes indicate the deficiency of *qi* and blood in the Gallbladder Meridian. Wrinkles under the outer corners of the eyes indicate muscle weakness in the upper limbs, muscle strain in the neck and shoulders, or frozen shoulder.

Facial Beauty *Gua Sha*

1. Apply facial *gua sha* cream. Use the corner of the scraper to scrape the Tongziliao and Taiyang acupoints on the outer corner of the eye respectively with the flat-pressing and kneading method, focusing on the wrinkled parts. Gently knead each part 5 times.

2. Use the flat-scraping method to scrape the wrinkled parts at the corners of the eyes slowly 5 to 10 times from the inside to the outside top, until the skin is slightly hot and flushed.

3. For those with wrinkles at the corners of the eyes and sagging, use the flat-scraping method to apply a pressing force into the muscles, starting from the Tongziliao acupoint and the upper limb area respectively, and scrape obliquely outward and upward to the edge of the hairline. Scrape each part 5 times.

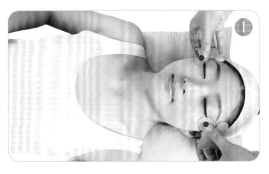
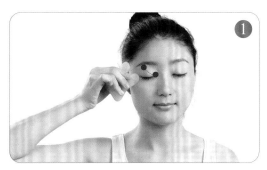
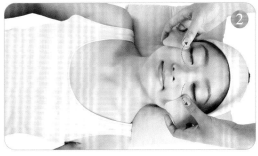
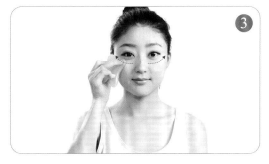

Consolidating *Gua Sha* on the Head and Neck

Put the scraper vertically on the edge of the hairline above the ear, and scrape both sides of the head from front to back around the ear. Then, use the single-angle method to scrape the Fengchi and Anmian acupoints on the neck.

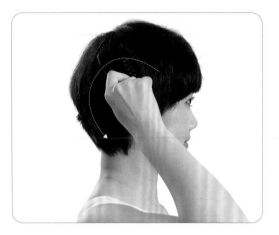

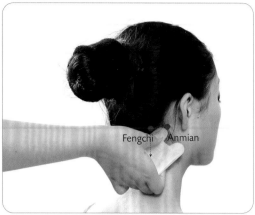

Fengchi   Anmian

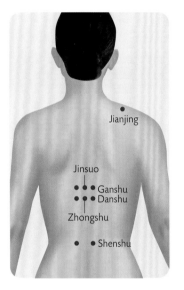

Jianjing

Jinsuo
Ganshu
Danshu
Zhongshu

Shenshu

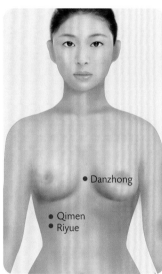

Danzhong

Qimen
Riyue

Whole-Body *Gua Sha* and Conditioning

1. Use the surface-scraping method to scrape the Jinsuo, Zhongshu, Ganshu, and Danshu acupoints on the back from top to bottom.

2. Use the surface-scraping method to scrape the Jianjing points on both sides of the shoulder from the inside to the outside.

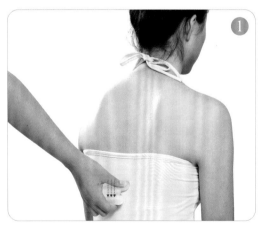

❶

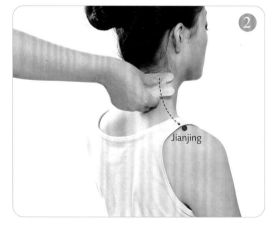

❷

Jianjing

3. Scrape the Danzhong acupoint on the chest from top to bottom with the single-angle method. Scrape the Qimen and Riyue acupoints on the abdomen from the inside to the outside with the flat-scraping method.

4. Use the surface-scraping method to scrape the Waiguan acupoint on the upper limbs from top to bottom. Scrape the Yanglingquan acupoint to the Waiqiu acupoint on both sides of the lower limbs from top to bottom with the surface-scraping method.

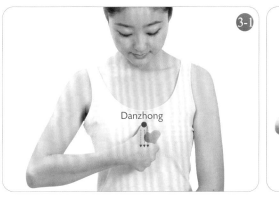

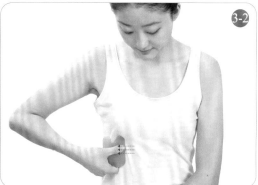

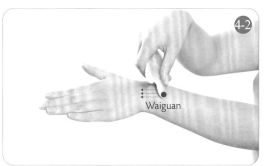

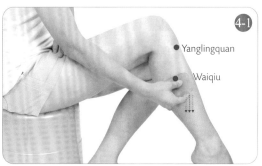

Expert Tip: The Relationships among Physiological Rhythms, Beauty, and Haircare

According to the physiological rhythms of the human body in the *Inner Canon of the Yellow Emperor*, significant physiological changes occur every 7 years for women and every 8 years for men. According to the *Inner Canon of the Yellow Emperor*, at the age of 42 for women and 48 for men, the *yang qi* in the body begins to fail, and gray hair begins to appear on the head. The earliest place where gray hair often appears is at the Taiyang acupoints, which is where the Gallbladder Meridian runs, starting from the outer corner of the eyes, along the sides of the head and down towards the side of the body. If there is a deficiency of *yang qi* in liver and gallbladder, the blood and *qi* will not come through. This leads to wrinkles, as well as early gray hair. Toning the liver and gallbladder *qi* and blood and unblocking the Gallbladder Meridian can help us improve these unattractive factors. In addition to performing facial *gua sha*, you can also use a scraping comb often, along the circulation of the Gallbladder Meridian, combing the hair and scraping the neck. This will unblock the *qi* and blood, reduce wrinkles, make your hair shiny, prevent cervical spondylosis, and tone your neck.

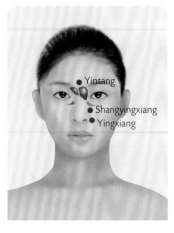

Wrinkles in the Middle of the Nose Bridge

Small crossed wrinkles and longitudinal wrinkles in the middle of the bridge of the nose are symptoms of deficiencies in the liver blood and liver and kidney *qi*. Most cases have liver and kidney deficiency and back pain, and severe cases have spinal disorders.

Facial Beauty *Gua Sha*

1. Apply facial *gua sha* cream. Press and knead the Yintang acupoint 5 times with the flat-pressing and kneading method.

2. Use the flat-scraping method to scrape from top to bottom, from the base to the tip of the nose 5 times, focusing on the middle of the bridge of the nose. Use the double corners of the scraper to straddle the bridge of the nose; scrape from the base to the tip of the nose from bottom to top 5 times, focusing on the middle of the bridge of the nose.

3. Scrape the Shangyingxiang and Yingxiang points with the flat-pressing and kneading method.

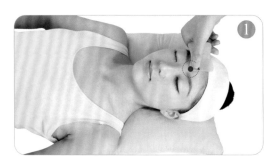

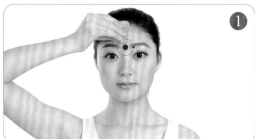

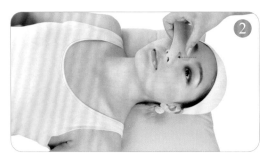

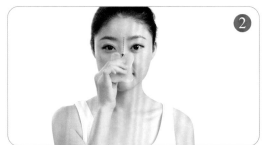

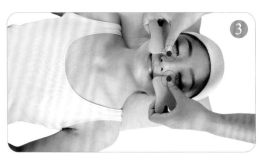

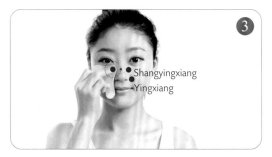

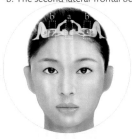

a: The mid-frontal belt
b. The second lateral-frontal belt

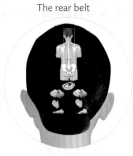

The rear belt

Consolidating *Gua Sha* on the Head, Hands, and Feet

1. Use the sharp-edge scraping method to scrape the mid-frontal belt, the second lateral-frontal belt, and the rear belt 5 to 10 times each.

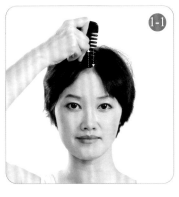

1-1

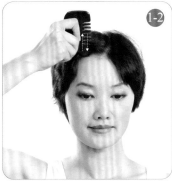

1-2

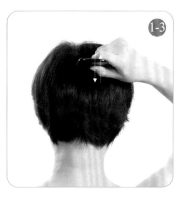

1-3

2. Scrape the liver and gallbladder area, the hypothenar area on the hands, the liver and gallbladder area, and the Yongquan acupoint in the soles with the flat-pressing and kneading method 5 to 10 times until the skin becomes slightly warm.

3. Scrape the lumbar area on the back of the hands and on the side of the feet 5 to 10 times with the pushing and scraping method.

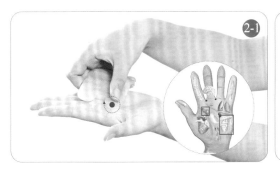

2-1

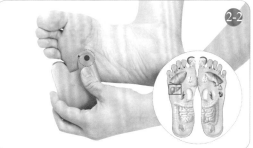

2-2

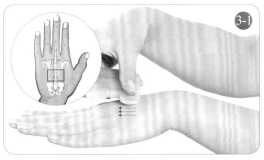

3-1

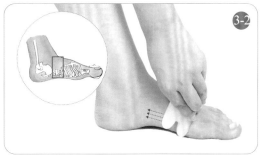

3-2

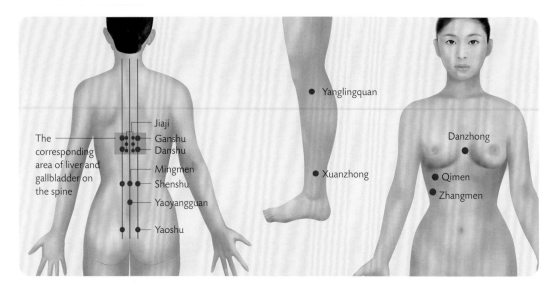

1. Scrape the corresponding area of liver and gallbladder on the spine: ① First use the surface-scraping method to scrape the Governor Vessel area between the 8th and 10th thoracic vertebrae. ② Use the dual-angle scraping method to scrape the Jiaji acupoints from top to bottom on both sides of the same horizontal section of the Governor Vessel. ③ Then, use the surface-scraping method to scrape the 3-cun wide area on both sides of the Governor Vessel from top to bottom. Scrape the Mingmen, Yaoshu, Yaoyangguan, Ganshu, Danshu, and Shenshu acupoints on the back from top to bottom with the surface-scraping method.

2. Scrape the Zhangmen and Qimen acupoints from inside to outside with the flat-scraping method.

3. Scrape the Yanglingquan and Xuanzhong acupoints on both lower limbs from top to bottom with the surface-scraping method.

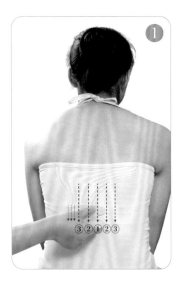

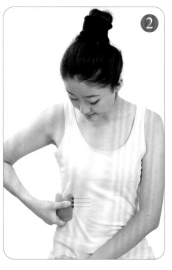

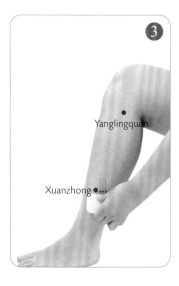

The spine is the pillar on which the human body stands, and is equivalent to the steel frame of a house. All of the important organs are under its protection. The health of the spine is very important throughout a person's life. Traditional Chinese medicine holds that the liver stores blood, the kidney stores essence, the essence produces marrow, and the marrow nourishes the bones. If the liver and kidneys are deficient, the muscles and bones will inevitably be weak. The middle of the bridge of the nose corresponds to the liver, and also to the spinal vertebrae in the middle and posterior region of the human body. If the liver blood is insufficient, the muscles and bones will be weak, and this part will lack luster or develop fine wrinkles. The curvature of the spine will also show subtle changes on the bridge of the nose. Therefore, to regulate fine wrinkles on the nose, in addition to performing facial *gua sha*, it is also necessary to deal with the liver and kidney, addressing the root cause of deficiencies.

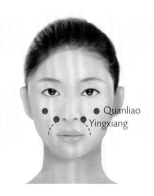

Loose Skin on the Cheek Areas and Nasolabial Folds

Loose skin in the cheek area and deep nasolabial folds is a sign of heart and spleen deficiency.

Facial Beauty *Gua Sha*

1. Apply facial *gua sha* cream, apply upward and outward pressure to massage the Yingxiang acupoint 5 times using the flat-pressing and kneading method.

2. Use the long arc edge of the scraper to push and scrape the Quanliao acupoint from the bottom to the top; find and scrape the positive reaction points 5 to 10 times.

3. Place the long arc edge of the scraper obliquely under the Yingxiang acupoint and the Quanliao acupoint, press downward to reach the deep part of the muscle, and push outward and upward to scrape the nasolabial folds.

4. Scrape the Quanliao acupoint and two cheek areas with the kneading and scraping method.

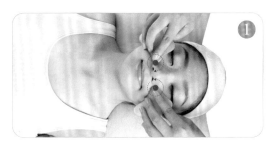

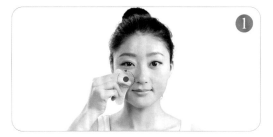

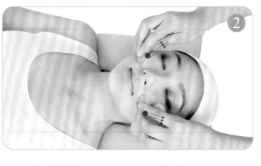

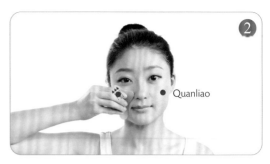

Quanliao

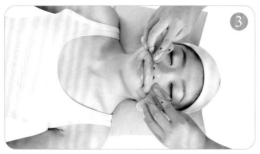

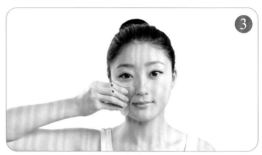

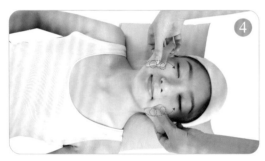

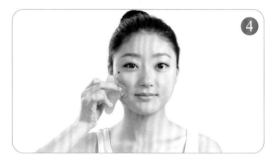

Consolidating *Gua Sha* on the Head, Hands, and Feet

1. Use the sharp-edge scraping method to scrape the first lateral-frontal belt, the second lateral-frontal belt on both sides, and the middle one-third area of the frontal belt of the head top.

    2. Scrape the whole palm with the surface-scraping method, focusing on the heart area of the thenar and the stomach area in the palm.

    3. Use the surface-scraping method to scrape the entire sole of the foot, focusing on the areas of the heart, stomach, and intestines.

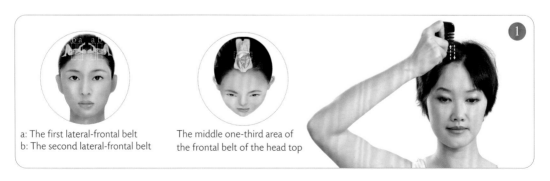

a: The first lateral-frontal belt
b: The second lateral-frontal belt

The middle one-third area of the frontal belt of the head top

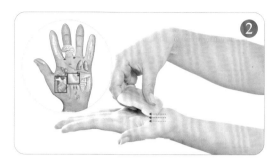
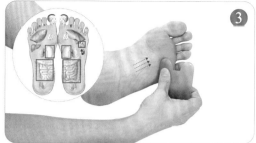

Whole-Body *Gua Sha* and Conditioning

1. Scrape the Xinshu, Pishu, Weishu, and Dachangshu acupoints on the back from top to bottom with the surface-scraping method.

    2. Scrape the projection area of spleen and pancreas on the body surface from the center to the left along the direction of the ribs with the flat-scraping method, or scrape 10 to 15 times through clothing until local heat is produced.

    3. Scrape the Danzhong, Zhongwan, and Xiawan acupoints from top to bottom with the surface-scraping method.

    4. Press and knead the Neiguan acupoint on the upper limbs and the Zusanli acupoint on the lower limbs with the flat-pressing and kneading method.

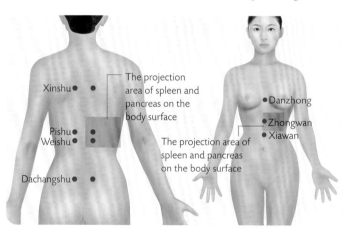
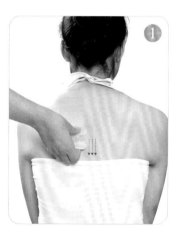

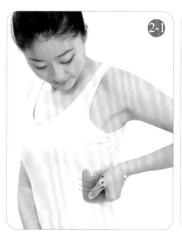
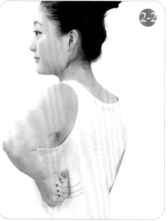
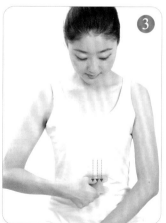

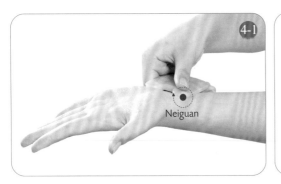

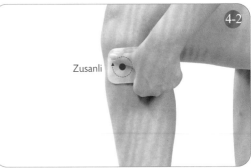

Skin wrinkles and loss of subcutaneous muscle elasticity can cause skin sagging. The loss of skin elasticity is closely related to insufficient access to cellular nutrition. Traditional Chinese medicine holds that the spleen dominates the muscles. If the spleen and stomach function well, they can provide adequate nutrition for the muscles. The skin will be elastic and firm, and the face will look younger than peers. Conversely, if the function of the spleen and stomach is not good, the muscles will become less elastic and relax prematurely. Loose skin on the cheek areas can deepen nasolabial folds, which is related to a deficiency of spleen and stomach *qi*, combined with overthinking and depletion of heart *qi*.

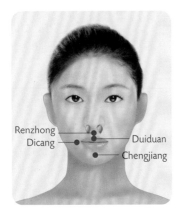

Upper and Lower Lip Wrinkles

Small wrinkles on the upper and lower lips and corners of the mouth are signs of spleen-stomach *qi* deficiency. Wrinkles on the upper lip are also symptoms of large intestine *qi* deficiency, ovarian atrophy, and sexual dysfunction.

Facial Beauty *Gua Sha*

1. Apply the facial *gua sha* cream, and use the corner of the scraper to massage the Renzhong acupoint and the bladder and ovary area in turn with the flat-pressing and kneading method.

2. Scrape the Dicang acupoint using the flat-pressing and kneading method with upward force.

3. Scrape the Chengjiang acupoint using the flat-pressing and kneading method.

4. Place the edge of the scraper flat on the Renzhong and Duiduan acupoints, scrape outward from the points to the Dicang acupoint with the flat-scraping method, and press the Dicang acupoint with upward pressure.

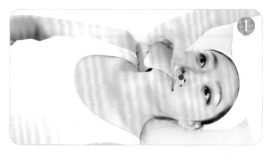

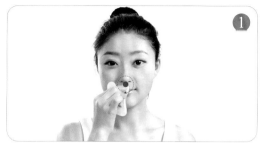

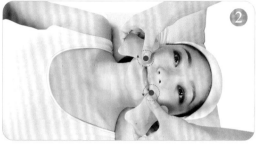

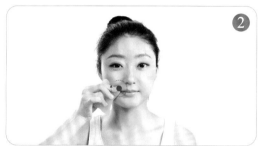

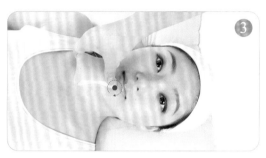

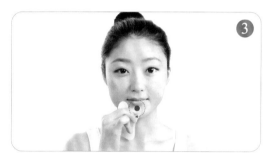

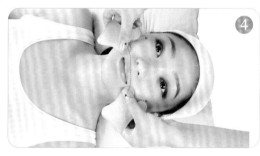

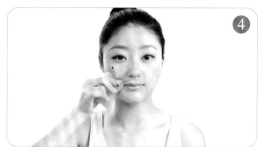

Consolidating *Gua Sha* on the Head, Hands, and Feet

1. Scrape the mid-frontal belt and the rear one-third area of the frontal belt of the head top.

    2. Scrape the hypothenar of the palm with the flat-pressing and kneading method, and scrape the inner and outer sides of the heel corresponding to the gonad area with the pushing and scraping method.

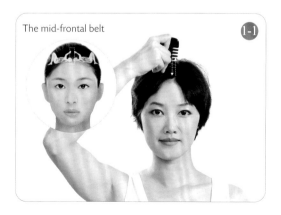

The mid-frontal belt

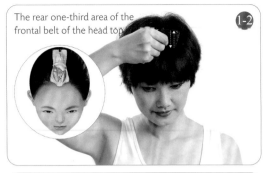

The rear one-third area of the frontal belt of the head top

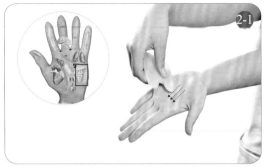

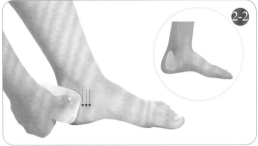

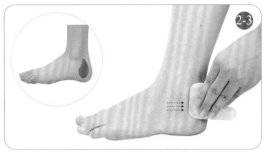

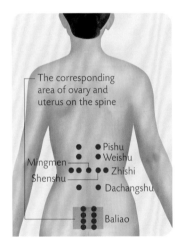

The corresponding area of ovary and uterus on the spine

Mingmen
Shenshu

Pishu
Weishu
Zhishi
Dachangshu

Baliao

Whole-Body *Gua Sha* and Conditioning

1. Scrape the Mingmen, Pishu, Weishu, Shenshu, Zhishi, and Dachangshu acupoints on the back from top to bottom with the surface-scraping method.

2. Scrape the corresponding area of the ovary and uterus on the spine, first scrape the Governor Vessel in the middle of the sacral vertebrae with the surface-scraping method, then scrape both sides of the Baliao acupoints at the same time with the double-angle scraping method, and scrape a 3-cun wide area on both sides of the spine with the surface-scraping method.

3. Scrape the Hegu and Neiguan acupoints on the hands with the flat-pressing and kneading method. Scrape the Zusanli, Sanyinjiao, and Taixi acupoints on the lower limbs from top to bottom with the surface-scraping method.

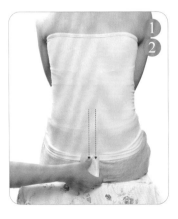

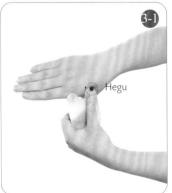

Hegu

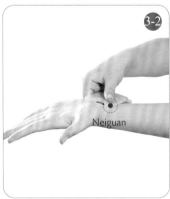

Neiguan

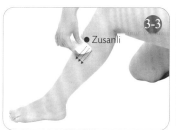

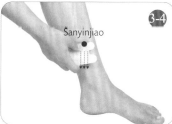

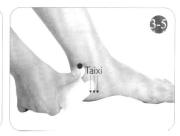

Expert tips: Improve the Spleen and Kidneys to Alleviate Wrinkles on the Mouth and Lips

Wrinkles on the upper and lower lips and at the corners of the mouth are a sign of weakened spleen and kidney function and reproductive function. This is because the mouth and lips are the external orifices of the spleen and the ultimate acupoint of the Conception Vessel and Governor Vessel, which both start from the uterus and are closely related to the function of the reproductive organs. In the biological holographic theory, the skin on the upper lip corresponds to the uterus and ovaries for women and the prostate for men. The appearance of wrinkles around the mouth means a deficiency of kidney essence, a weakening of reproductive function, and a deficiency of spleen and stomach *qi*, which are signs that both innate and acquired *qi* are insufficient. Wrinkles in the upper lip area generally deepen with age. If wrinkles appear prematurely on the upper and lower lip, it is a sign of premature aging. This is the reason why the spleen and kidney should be tonified to alleviate wrinkles around the mouth.

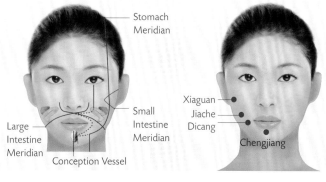

Wrinkles on the Lower Jaw

Transverse wrinkles in the middle of the lower jaw are a sign of kidney deficiency, lower back pain, or hemorrhoids. Wrinkles and sagging on both sides of the lower jaw are symptoms of spleen *qi* deficiency, weakened digestive function, and weakness of the lower limbs.

Facial Beauty *Gua Sha*

1. Apply facial *gua sha* cream. First, press and knead the Chengjiang and Dicang acupoints 5 times each using the flat-pressing and kneading method, and then scrape the Chengjiang acupoint to the Jiache acupoint and the Xiaguan acupoint with the pushing and scraping method along the circulation line of the Stomach Meridian, looking for and

focusing on the positive reaction points with 5 to 10 times.

2. Use the pushing and scraping method to scrape the lower limb area, looking for and focusing on the positive reaction points 5 to 10 times.

3. Use the pushing and scraping method to scrape the Conception Vessel with the groove at the corner of the scraper, and scrape the area of Stomach Meridian, Large Intestine Meridian, and Small Intestine Meridian on both sides.

4. Scrape the lower limb area with the kneading and scraping method in an upward arc.

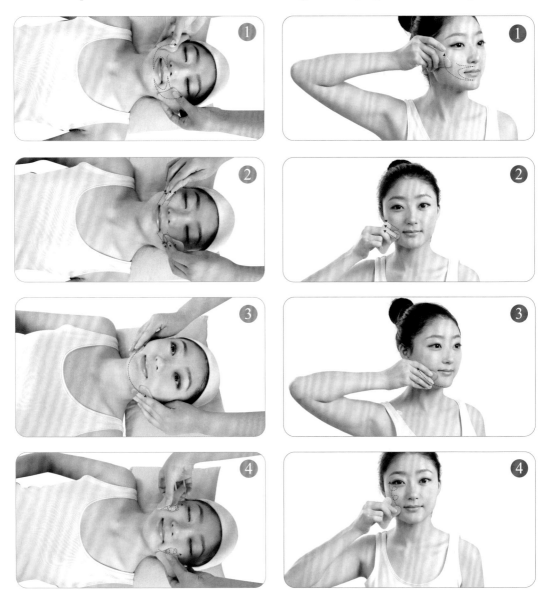

Consolidating *Gua Sha* on the Head, Hands, and Feet

1. Use the sharp-edge scraping method to scrape the third lateral-frontal belt on both sides of the head, the middle one-third area of the frontal belt of the head top, and the rear one-third area of the frontal belt of the head top.

2. Use the flat-scraping method to scrape the kidney area and the uterus area of the hands and feet, and scrape the index finger and little finger with the groove of the scraper.

3. Scrape the heel and the inner and outer sides of the heel corresponding to the gonad areas with the pushing and scraping method.

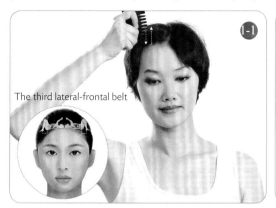

The third lateral-frontal belt

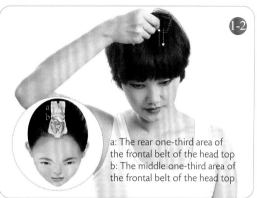

a: The rear one-third area of the frontal belt of the head top
b: The middle one-third area of the frontal belt of the head top

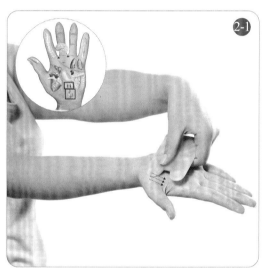

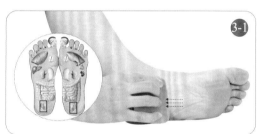

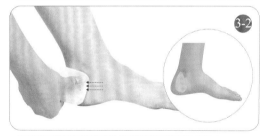

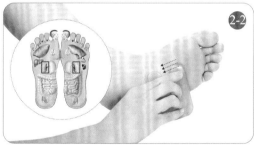

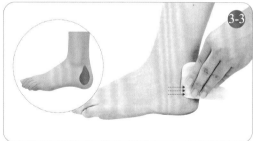

Whole-Body *Gua Sha* and Conditioning

1. Scrape the Mingmen, Pishu, Weishu, and Shenshu acupoints on the back from top to bottom with the surface-scraping method.

2. Scrape the corresponding area of ovary and uterus on the spine: ① Scrape the Governor Vessel in the middle of the 2nd to 4th sacral vertebrae with the surface-scraping

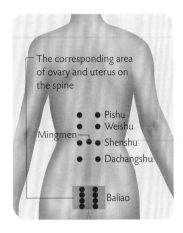

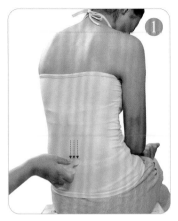

The corresponding area of ovary and uterus on the spine

Pishu
Weishu
Mingmen — Shenshu
Dachangshu

Baliao

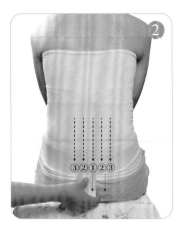

Yanglingquan

method. ② Use the double-angle scraping method to scrape the Baliao acupoints on both sides at the same time. ③ Scrape the 3-cun wide range on both sides of the sacral vertebrae with the surface-scraping method.

3. Scrape the Zusanli and Yanglingquan acupoints on the lower limbs from top to bottom with the surface-scraping method.

Expert Tips: Nourishing the Kidneys for Beauty and Fitness

Abundant kidney *qi* can work to regulate the water in the body, and any excess water will be discharged timely. The *Inner Canon of the Yellow Emperor* says that a woman's kidney *qi* gradually declines from the age of 35. When her kidney *qi* fails, water cannot be discharged in a timely manner, which can cause abdominal obesity or bloating. Kidney *qi* can be supplemented to reduce waist circumference without losing weight. This is because the kidneys govern the bones. If the kidneys are working well, the bone density will increase. Even if no weight is lost, you will develop healthy curves. The essence of the kidney is reflected in the hair. When the kidney *qi* is flourishing, the hair will be thick and strongly colored; if the kidney *qi* is insufficient, the hair will be dry and brittle. People with sufficient kidney *qi* have a rosy complexion and soft skin.

The lower jaw area corresponds to the lower *jiao*. Whether the kidney *qi* is sufficient is reflected in this area, most obviously in the mouth and lips. Wrinkles around the mouth and jaw are signs of kidney *qi* deficiency. Kidney deficiency can lead to a sore lower back and weak knees, a lack of *qi* in the lower limbs, and blood deficiency. In addition to warming and tonifying kidney *yang*, physical exercise should also be intensified. Increasing the strength of the lower limbs muscles will help slow down wrinkles in this area.

Diet Therapy and Skin Care

Nucleic acid is a "life information" substance that can delay aging and strengthen and beautify the skin. Some studies have shown that after 4 weeks, women who consume 800 mg of nucleic acid daily will see an obvious reduction in wrinkles, a fading of age spots, and relief from rough and dry skin. Nucleic acid-rich foods include fish, shrimp, yeast, mushrooms, black fungus, and pollen. Taking vitamin C or eating fresh fruit and vegetables at the same time is conducive to the absorption of nucleic acids.

You should also consume yogurt regularly. The vitamin C contained in it can reduce the deposition of melanin in the body, while the calcium, magnesium, potassium, sodium and other minerals and trace elements can reduce pigmentation and relieve wrinkles. Long-term consumption of yogurt can increase skin elasticity and lessen pigmentation.

Food Therapy Recipe

Winter melon and meatball soup: Winter melon is rich in vitamins and fatty acids. Eaten regularly, it can help you lose weight and reduce swelling, moisturize, whiten your skin, and resist the generation of wrinkles in the early stages, leaving skin soft and smooth.

Peel and clean 500 grams of winter melon, and cut into small cubes. Mince 250 grams of pork, add salt and flour, and knead into meatballs. When kneading the meatballs, add a small amount of cornstarch to make them firm, maintain their shape, and make them less likely to break apart during cooking.

Place the meatballs and seasonings in a saucepan and simmer over a low heat with a good amount of clean water for 20 minutes, then add the winter melon and cook over low heat for 15 minutes.

Homemade Wrinkle-Reducing Masks

• Cucumber and honey mask: 1 fresh cucumber, 1 spoonful of honey. Wash and blend the cucumber. Add the honey and mix evenly. Coat your face, and leave on for 20 to 30 minutes, then wash off with water. Or, cut the cucumber into thin slices, dip them in honey, and paste onto your face every morning and evening. In addition to its anti-wrinkle properties, this mask also nourishes the skin and enhances elasticity.

• Egg and honey mask: 1 egg, 1 spoonful of honey. Mix egg white and honey, then spread it evenly on the forehead and eye wrinkles. Close your eyes and rest, and wait for it to dry naturally. After 30 minutes, wash it off with water. Use 2 to 3 times a week to moisturize, reduce wrinkles, and delay aging.

• Orange and honey mask: 1 orange, 1 spoonful of honey. Wash the orange and mash it in a bowl, including the skin. Add honey and mix well. Refrigerate for 2 to 3 hours before use. Apply to wrinkles every morning and evening, and wash off with water after about 20 minutes. This method gets rid of wrinkles and lubricates the skin.

• Tomato and honey mask: 1 tomato, an appropriate amount of honey. Wash and chop the tomatoes. Squeeze into juice, add the honey, and blend evenly. Coat the face, and wash off with water when it has dried. Apply once in the morning and once in the evening, for 20 to 30 minutes each time, to moisturize and remove wrinkles.

CHAPTER SIX
Eliminating Acne

Acne is a common chronic inflammatory skin disease of hair follicles and sebaceous glands. It mainly occurs in people with strong oil secretion, and is related to a poor diet, excessive mental stress, endocrine disorders, and constipation. The location and nature of the disorder of *qi* and blood in the viscera are different, which determines the location and form of facial acne. Therefore, scraping to treat facial acne is not scraping directly on the acne on the face, but rather scraping the meridians and holographic acupoints below the face to regulate the *qi* and blood of the viscera, meridians, so as to achieve the balance of *yin* and *yang*, and *qi* and blood in the internal environment.

Note: Some acupoints involved in this book are distributed symmetrically on both sides of the body. When conducting facial *gua sha*, except for a few acupoints that require one-sided scraping, the rest are all symmetrical acupoints on both sides of the body by default.

Key Points of the Technique

1. Facial acne is an external manifestation of heat and fire in the body. *Gua Sha* regulates the functions of the viscera, blood, and meridians to remove it.

2. According to the location of facial acne, the corresponding meridian and viscera on the body to be scraped can be determined; according to the form of acne, the method of tonifying and purgative (high pressure and fast speed) can be determined.

3. Acne that is small in shape, light in color, and low in number is due to flaring up of deficient fire. Scrape with the tonifying method, the scraping area should be limited, and the scraping time should be short. Once a small number of *sha* are scraped out, the scraping should be stopped so as not to damage the vital *qi*. Acne that is large in shape, bright red in color, and high in number is caused by excess fire, and can be scraped with the uniform reinforcing-reducing method (medium pressure, moderate speed), scraping each part until no new *sha* appear.

4. After the acne has improved and subsided from scraping and conditioning, use the *gua sha* method for daily beauty, and use the pushing and scraping method on the acne-prone parts of the face; find and focus on the positive reaction points, and dredge the meridians to help prevent recurrence. Use flat-scraping method to speed up the healing of acne marks.

Acne All over the Face

In principle, facial *gua sha* is not used for acne removal, and the acne-prone areas should not be scraped. Directly scraping will aggravate skin infection.

Gua Sha on the Head, Neck, Hands, and Feet
1. Use a scraping comb to scrape the top, back, and lateral head with the surface-scraping method.

2. Use the surface-scraping method to scrape the middle and sides of the front of the neck from top to bottom.

3. Scrape the corresponding area of head and face on the spine. ① First use the surface-scraping to scrape the region of Governor Vessel on the 1st to 7th cervical vertebrae. ② Use the dual-angle scraping method to scrape the Bladder Meridian on both sides of the cervical spine from top to bottom.

4. Use the flat-pressing and kneading method to scrape the Hegu acupoint. Use the surface-scraping method to scrape the thenar and hypothenar in the palm, the stomach area and the intestine area in the sole.

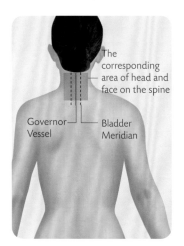

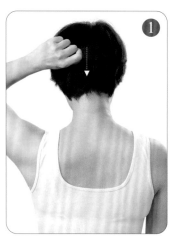

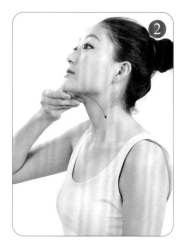

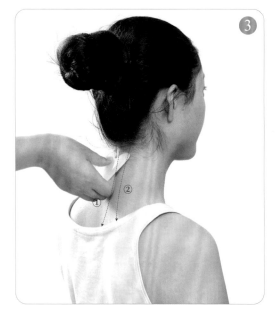

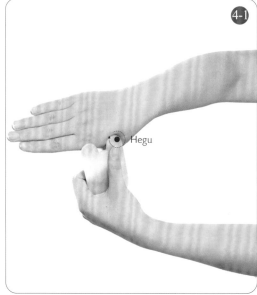

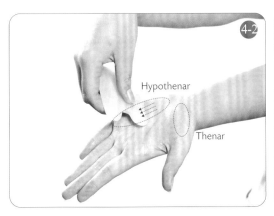

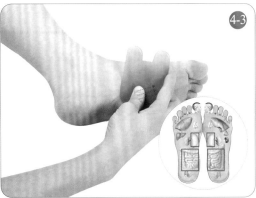

Whole-Body *Gua Sha* and Conditioning

1. Use the surface-scraping method to scrape the Dazhui, Jiaji, Feishu, Pishu, Danshu, Weishu, Sanjiaoshu, and Dachangshu acupoints.

    2. Use the surface-scraping method to scrape the Quchi and Hegu acupoints on the upper limbs and the Fenglong acupoints on the lower limbs from bottom to top.

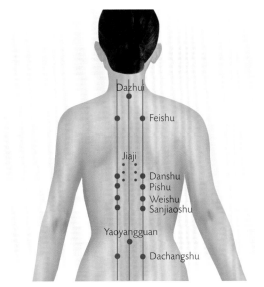

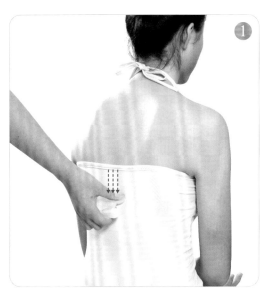

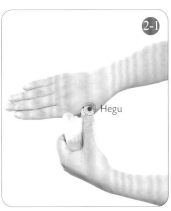

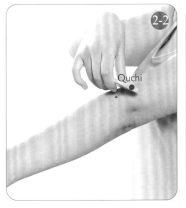

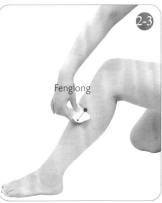

Acne in the Middle of the Forehead

The middle of the forehead up to the anterior hairline and down to between the eyebrows is the area where the Governor Vessel and the Bladder Meridian run. It is also a holographic

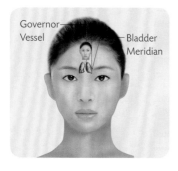

Governor Vessel

Bladder Meridian

acupoint area for the brain, the lung and the throat. Acne that is light in color, in large quantity and recurring in this area, is indicative of overuse of the brain and a flare-up of deficient fire in the lungs and kidneys. Painful, recurring acne between the eyebrows that is light in color and not obvious, is associated with deficient fire in the Lung Meridian, and is often accompanied by shortness of breath, dry mouth, sore throat, or chronic pharyngitis.

Gua Sha on the Head and Neck

1. Use the sharp-edge scraping method to scrape the mid-frontal belt and use a scraping comb to scrape the rear belt on the top of the head and the back of the head with the surface-scraping method.

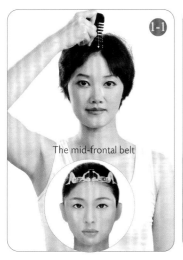

The mid-frontal belt

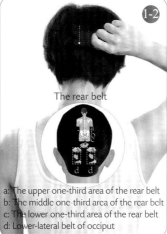

The rear belt

a: The upper one-third area of the rear belt
b: The middle one-third area of the rear belt
c: The lower one-third area of the rear belt
d: Lower-lateral belt of occiput

2. Scrape the Governor Vessel on the neck with the surface-scraping method, and scrape the Bladder Meridian area on both sides of the neck with the dual-angle scraping method.

3. Use the surface-scraping method to scrape the projection area of throat on the anterior neck from top to bottom.

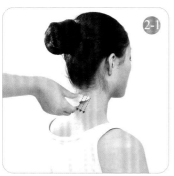

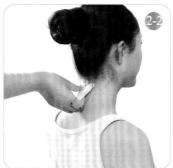

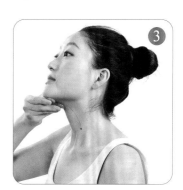

Whole-Body *Gua Sha* and Conditioning

1. Use the surface-scraping method to scrape the Dazhui, Feishu, and Shenshu acupoints from top to bottom.

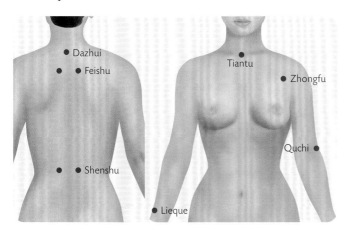

Dazhui
Feishu
Tiantu
Zhongfu
Quchi
Shenshu
Lieque

2. Use the single-angle scraping method to scrape the Tiantu and Zhongfu acupoints on the chest from top to bottom.

3. Use the surface-scraping method to scrape the Quchi and Lieque acupoints on the upper limbs from top to bottom.

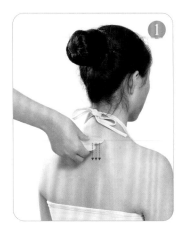
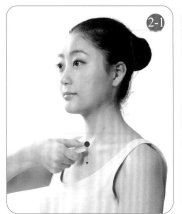
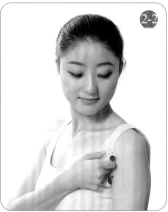
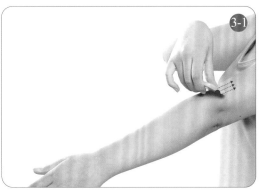
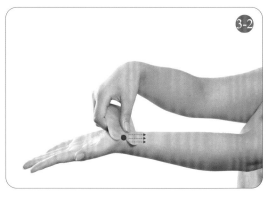

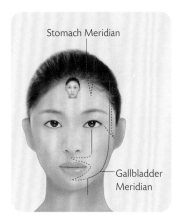

Stomach Meridian

Gallbladder Meridian

Acne on the Lateral Sides of the Forehead

The forehead is the holographic acupoint area corresponding to the brain, and the outer side of the forehead is the circulation area for the Gallbladder Meridian and the Stomach Meridian. Acne here indicates heat exuberance in the stomach, liver, and gallbladder, mostly due to excessive use of the brain, high mental stress, liver dysfunction, and weakened liver detoxification function. It is often accompanied by anxiety, insomnia, and a bitter taste in the mouth.

Gua Sha on the Head and Neck

1. Use a scraping comb to scrape the side of the head with the surface-scraping method. Scrape the mid-frontal belt with the sharp-edge scraping method. The method is the same as on page 124 for acne in the middle of the forehead.

2. Use the surface-scraping method to scrape the Fengfu acupoint to the Dazhui acupoint on the neck (the same method as for acne in the middle of the forehead.) At the same time, use the single-angle scraping method to scrape the Fengchi acupoint on the neck and the Gallbladder Meridian area on both sides of the neck.

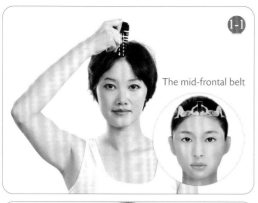

The mid-frontal belt

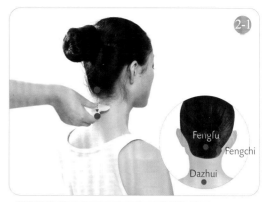

Fengfu
Fengchi
Dazhui

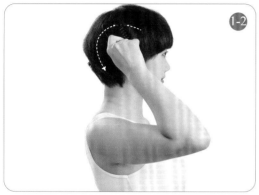

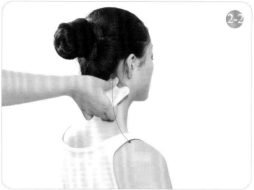

Whole-Body *Gua Sha* and Conditioning

1. Use the surface-scraping method to scrape the Dazhui, Ganshu, Danshu, and Weishu acupoints from top to bottom.

2. Use the surface-scraping method to scrape the Jianjing acupoint on the shoulder from the inside out.

3. Use the surface-scraping method to scrape the Waiguan and Zhigou acupoints on the upper limbs from top to bottom.

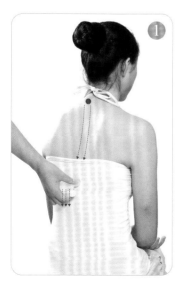

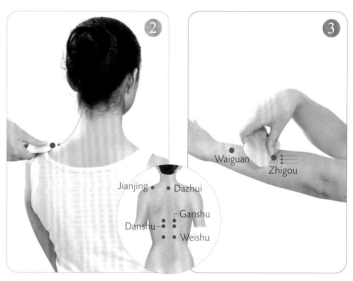

Jianjing   Dazhui

Ganshu

Danshu   Weishu

Waiguan
Zhigou

The human body has a sympathetic nervous system and a parasympathetic nervous system. The activity of the sympathetic nervous system mainly meets the physiological needs of the body in a state of tension. Stimulation of the sympathetic nerves can cause vasoconstriction of the abdominal viscera and peripheral skin, and can strengthen and accelerate the heartbeat, hypermetabolism, and constriction of the pupils, as well as increasing the working ability of tired muscles. The main function of the parasympathetic nerve is to dilate the pupils, slow the heartbeat, dilate blood vessels in the skin and viscera, constrict small bronchi, strengthen gastrointestinal motility, relax the sphincter, and increase saliva secretion.

TCM holds that overthinking, stress, and a bad mood can create excessive internal heat because you are constantly using your sympathetic nervous system, tricking your body into thinking that you are in a state of danger or emergency, instead of invoking the parasympathetic nervous system constantly to soothe and relax you. *Gua Sha* can help you solve problems temporarily, but if you don't fundamentally adjust your mentality, acne will recur.

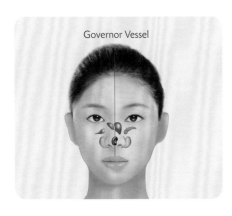

Governor Vessel

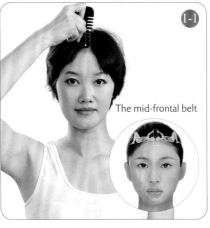

The mid-frontal belt

Acne on the Nose

The middle of the nose is the area where the Governor Vessel runs, and corresponds to the holographic area of the liver, gallbladder, and pancreas. The tip and wings of the nose correspond to the holographic area of the spleen and stomach. Among the five sense organs, the nose is also the lung orifice. Acne on the tip and wings of the nose indicates heat in the spleen, stomach, and lungs, and excessive heat in the stomach, often accompanied by a strong appetite, a preference for sweet, fatty, and rich-flavored foods, and an excessive intake of fat; redness of the nose is related to endocrine disorders, and severe cases will lead to rosacea. This indicates damp heat in the spleen and stomach or excessive drinking, as well as increased blood pressure, blood lipids, and blood sugar.

Gua Sha on the Head and Neck

1. Use the sharp-edge scraping method to scrape

the mid-frontal belt. Use a scraping comb to scrape the top and back of the head with the surface-scraping method.

2. Use the surface-scraping method to scrape the Fengfu acupoint to the Dazhui acupoint on the neck, and use the dual-angle scraping method to scrape the Bladder Meridian area on both sides of the neck.

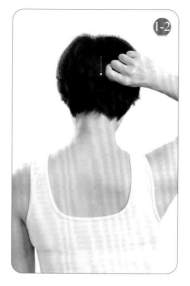

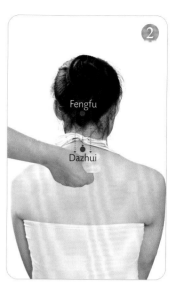

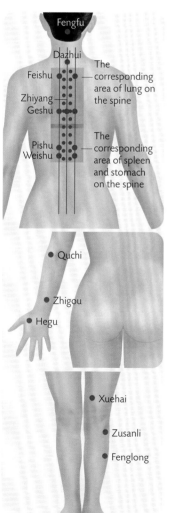

Whole-Body *Gua Sha* and Conditioning

1. Use the surface-scraping method to scrape the corresponding areas of the lung, spleen, and stomach on the spine. ① Use the surface-scraping method to scrape the Governor Vessel in the middle of the 1st to 9th and 8th to 12th thoracic vertebrae from top to bottom. ② Use the dual-angle method to scrape the Jiaji acupoints from top to bottom on both sides of the same horizontal section of the Governor Vessel. ③ Use the surface-scraping method to scrape the 3-cun wide area on both sides of the Governor Vessel from top to bottom. Focus on scraping the Dazhui acupoint to the Zhiyang, Feishu, Geshu, Pishu, and Weishu acupoints.

2. Use the surface-scraping the to scrape the Quchi, Zhigou, and Hegu acupoints on the upper limbs from top to bottom, and scrape the Zusanli acupoint to the Fenglong and Xuehai acupoints on the lower limbs from top to bottom.

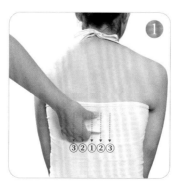

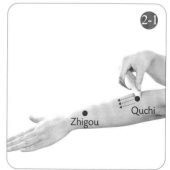

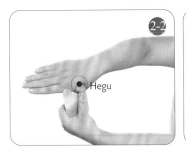

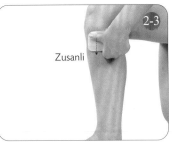

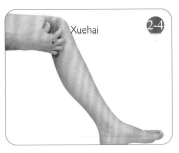

Zusanli

Hegu

Xuehai

Expert Tips: An Improper Diet Can Create "Fire"

We have already discussed the heat exuberance of the six *fu* organs, the deficiency-heat caused by a *yin* deficiency of the lungs and kidneys, and the stagnated heat caused by emotional discomfort. There is also food heat, which is caused by over-eating or eating sweet, fatty, and rich-flavored foods that cannot be digested.

TCM beauty and health encourages a light diet. Women who are interested in beauty generally eat less food with high fat content such as fatty meat, but it is difficult to avoid food with rich flavors. Spicy hot pot, which many women enjoy, are particularly rich-flavored. It is the same with sweet, fatty dishes such as cake and ice cream. If you don't limit your intake of these foods, you will be vulnerable to internal heat.

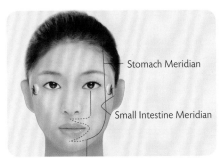

Stomach Meridian

Small Intestine Meridian

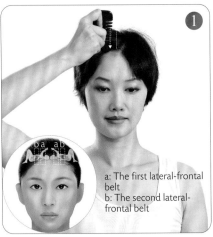

a: The first lateral-frontal belt
b: The second lateral-frontal belt

Acne on the Cheek Areas

The two cheek areas are the parts where the Small Intestine Meridian runs. They are also the holographic acupoint areas corresponding to the large intestine and the small intestine. The Stomach Meridian runs through the inner and outer sides of the two cheek areas, and the outer sides are the holographic acupoint areas corresponding to the kidneys. Acne on the cheeks indicates heat accumulation in the small intestine and stomach, leading to a flare-up of heart fire. It is mostly related to over-eating sweet, fatty, and spicy food, not drinking enough water, or excessive mental stress, and is often accompanied by depression or irritability.

Gua Sha on the Head, Hands, and Feet

1. Use the sharp-edge scraping method to scrape the first lateral-frontal belt and the second lateral-

frontal belt on both sides of the head.

2. Use the surface-scraping method to scrape the holographic areas of the heart and the large and small intestines on the hands and feet.

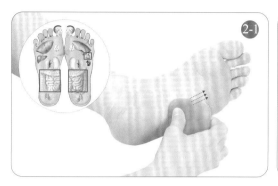

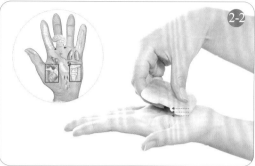

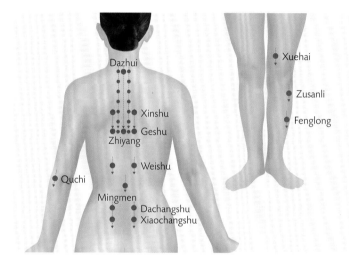

Whole-Body *Gua Sha* and Conditioning

1. Use the surface-scraping method to scrape from the Dazhui acupoint to the Mingmen acupoint, the Xinshu acupoint to the Geshu, Weishu, Dachangshu, and Xiaochangshu acupoints on the back from top to bottom.

2. Use the dual-angle scraping method to scrape the bilateral Jiaji acupoints parallel to the section of Dazhui acupoint to the Zhiyang acupoint from top to bottom.

3. Use the surface-scraping method to scrape the Quchi acupoint on the upper limbs, and the Xuehai and Zusanli acupoints to the Fenglong acupoint on the lower limbs from top to bottom.

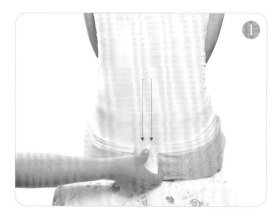

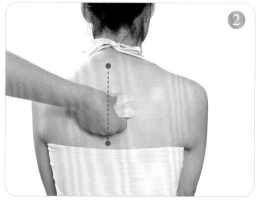

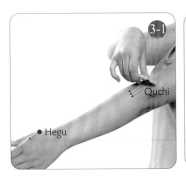
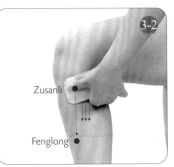
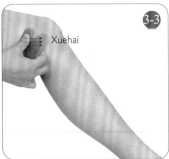

3-1 · Quchi · Hegu

3-2 · Zusanli · Fenglong

3-3 · Xuehai

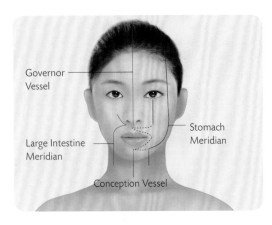

Governor Vessel

Large Intestine Meridian

Stomach Meridian

Conception Vessel

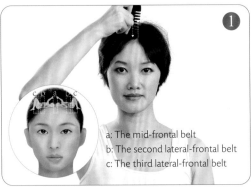

1

a: The mid-frontal belt
b: The second lateral-frontal belt
c: The third lateral-frontal belt

Acne around the Mouth

The lips are the circulation area of the Stomach Meridian, Large Intestine Meridian, and the Conception Vessel and Governor Vessel, and the mouth is the external orifice of the spleen. Acne around the mouth is often accompanied by a strong appetite, abdominal bloating, bad breath, thirst, constipation, yellow urine, and irregular menstruation, suggesting gastrointestinal heat exuberance, internal stagnation, and endocrine disorders and gynecological disorders in women with stubborn acne around the mouth.

Gua Sha on the Head, Hands, and Feet

1. Use the sharp-edge scraping method to scrape the mid-frontal belt, the second lateral-frontal belt and third lateral-frontal belt on both sides.

2. Use the surface-scraping method to scrape the stomach area, large intestine area of the hands and feet, and the gonad area on both sides of the heel.

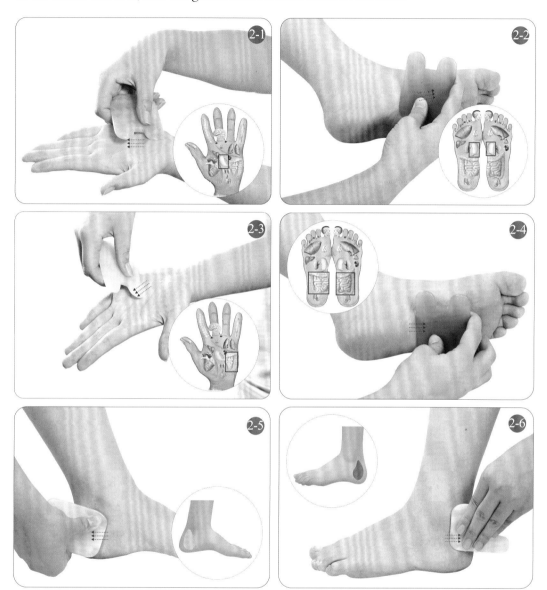

Whole-Body *Gua Sha* and Conditioning

1. Use the surface-scraping method to scrape the corresponding area of spleen and stomach on the spine. ① Use the surface-scraping method to scrape the Governor Vessel in the middle of the 8th to 12th thoracic vertebrae from top to bottom. ② Use the dual-angle scraping method to scrape the Jiaji acupoints from top to bottom on both sides of the same horizontal section of the Governor Vessel. ③ Use the surface-scraping method to scrape the 3-cun wide area on both sides of the Governor Vessel from top to bottom, and focus on scraping the Dazhui, Pishu, Weishu, and Dachangshu acupoints.

    2. Use the surface-scraping method to scrape the Zhongwan and Xiawan acupoints

on the abdomen from top to bottom.

3. Use the surface-scraping method to scrape the Quchi and Hegu acupoints on the upper limbs, and the Fenglong and Gongsun acupoints on the lower limbs from top to bottom.

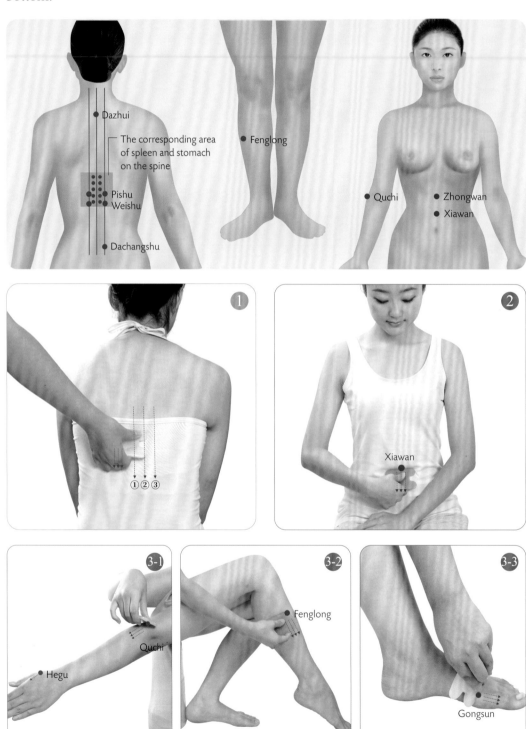

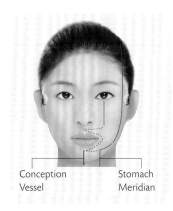

Conception
Vessel

Stomach
Meridian

Stubborn Acne in the Middle of the Lower Jaw

The lower jaw is the area where the Conception Vessel and Stomach Meridian flow. It is also a holographic acupoint area corresponding to the reproductive organs and kidneys. If acne occurs repeatedly, or if the skin of the lower jaw is dull and less lustrous, accompanied by coldness in the lower back, abdomen, and hands and feet, this suggests that the nature of acne is coldness in the lower *jiao*, resulting in a flare-up of deficient fire, which causes acne.

If the skin has excessive oil secretion, with frequently occurring acne that is dark red, accompanied by a preference for sweet, fatty food, with dark urine or uncomfortable bowel movement, this suggests acne caused by damp heat in the lower *jiao*.

Women with acne that worsens during the premenstrual period are suffering from endocrine disorders, often accompanied by symptoms of irregular menstruation. Acne that is stubborn and difficult to cure can be a sign of polycystic ovaries, and you should seek a further gynecological diagnosis at a hospital.

Gua Sha on the Head, Hands and Feet

1. Use the sharp-edge scraping method to scrape the mid-frontal belt and the third lateral-frontal belt on both sides.

2. Press and knead the gonad area on both sides of the heel with the flat-pressing and kneading method.

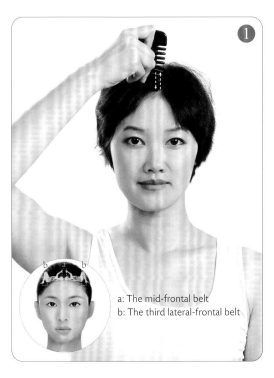

a: The mid-frontal belt
b: The third lateral-frontal belt

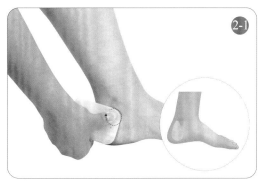

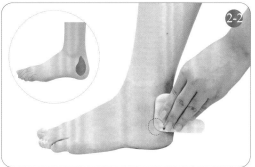

Whole-Body *Gua Sha* and Conditioning

1. Scrape the corresponding area of the reproductive organs in the lumbosacral region. ① Use the surface-scraping method to scrape the Governor Vessel in the middle of the 2nd to 4th sacral vertebrae. ② Use the dual-angle scraping method to scrape the Baliao acupoints on both sides at the same time. ③ Use the surface-scraping method to scrape the 3-cun wide area on both sides of the sacral vertebrae, focusing on the Shenshu and Baliao acupoints.

2. Use the surface-scraping method to scrape the projection area of the uterus and ovary on the body surface in the lower abdomen from top to bottom.

3. Use the surface-scraping method to scrape the Quchi acupoints on the upper limbs, and Fenglong, Taixi and Shuiquan acupoints on the lower limbs, from top to bottom.

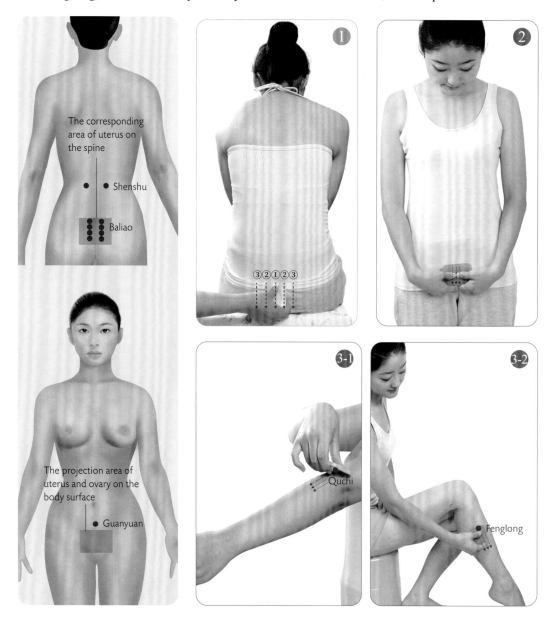

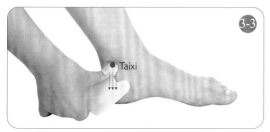

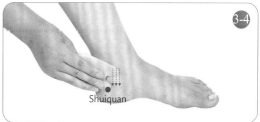

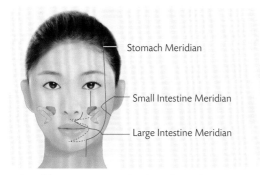

Stomach Meridian

Small Intestine Meridian

Large Intestine Meridian

Stubborn Acne on Both Sides of the Lower Jaw

Both sides of the lower jaw are where the Stomach Meridian, Large Intestine Meridian, and Small Intestine Meridian run. It is also the holographic acupoint area of the lower limbs, and mostly reflects the health status of the lower *jiao*. The causes of stubborn acne on both sides of the lower jaw are the most complicated. Acne with a large, reddish form and obvious inflammation is mostly due to excess heat; a small, light-colored form is mostly due to deficiency-heat; nodular cystic acne is mostly due to internal phlegm-dampness; oily skin with significant inflammation is mostly due to damp-heat; and acne with a dark red color and insignificant pain is mostly due to blood stasis. Damp-heat in the lower *jiao* is the most common, and there may be symptoms of yellow urine, heavy odor, sticky stools and uncomfortable bowel movement, heaviness and fatigue of the lower limbs. In women, leukorrhea is abundant and yellow in color.

Gua Sha **for the Head and Hands**

1. Use the sharp-edge scraping method to scrape the mid-frontal belt, the second lateral-frontal belt and the third lateral-frontal belt.

2. Scrape the thenar and hypothenar, and the kidney and bladder areas of the hand with the surface-scraping method.

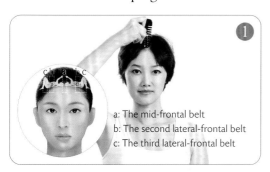

a: The mid-frontal belt
b: The second lateral-frontal belt
c: The third lateral-frontal belt

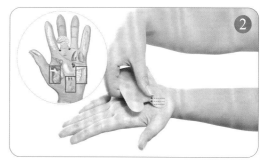

Whole-Body *Gua Sha* **and Conditioning**

1. Scrape the Weishu, Sanjiaoshu, Shenshu, Dachangshu, and Pangguangshu acupoints from top to bottom with the surface-scraping method.

2. Scrape the abdomen from the top downward from the Zhongzhu acupoint to the Qixue acupoint and from the Jianli acupoint to the Shuifen acupoint with the surface-scraping method.

3. Use the surface-scraping method to scrape the Quchi acupoints on the upper limbs, and the Fenglong, Taixi, and Shuiquan acupoints on the lower limbs from top to bottom.

4. For those with blood stasis, also scrape the Geshu acupoint on the back and the Xuehai acupoint on the lower limbs.

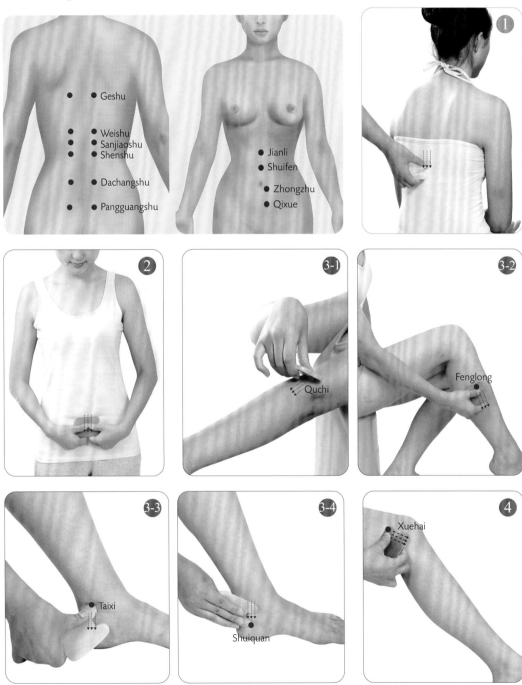

Diet Therapy and Skin Care

Keep your bowel movements smooth, drink plenty of water, take crude fiber or intestinal clearing and detoxification food, such as fruit, vegetables, whole grains, black fungus, algae, and starchy vegetables. Regular consumption of winter melon, red beans, and mung beans can prevent and treat skin infections.

Clean your skin carefully, and avoid alcohol and other irritating food, as well as sweet food and ingredients with a high fat content.

Mashing tomato, purslane, and cactus separately and applying any one of them on acne has a therapeutic effect.

Food Therapy Recipes

• Take 25 grams of mung beans, 25 grams of coix seed, and 10 grams of hawthorn. Wash, and add 500 grams of water. Soak for 30 minutes then bring to a boil. After boiling for a few minutes, turn off the heat. Do not remove the cover. Simmer for 15 minutes, and drink it as tea, 3 to 5 times a day. This is suitable for oily skin.

• Take an appropriate amount of small Chinese cabbage, celery, bitter gourd, bell pepper, lemon, apple, and mung beans. Boil the mung beans for 30 minutes, then filter the juice. Wash the cabbage, celery, bitter gourd, bell pepper, and apple separately, then cut into sections or pieces. Squeeze the juice, add mung bean juice, drip in lemon juice, and add honey to taste. Drink 1 to 2 times a day to clear heat, detoxify, and sterilize.

Homemade Face Mask for Acne Relief

• Anti-inflammatory aloe vera and cucumber mask: Both aloe vera and cucumber have anti-inflammatory effects. Buy fresh aloe vera, cut it into small pieces, and apply it to the affected area, and peel the cucumber and squeeze it into juice. Apply it to a freshly washed face and rinse it off after about 30 minutes. Drinking cucumber juice with honey is also very effective.

• Mung bean and bitter gourd mask: Wash the bitter gourd, mash it with its skin, then add honey, tea tree essential oil, and an appropriate amount of distilled water in turn. Mix well, and finally add the ground mung bean powder and mix again. Clean your face and apply the mask directly. After 15 to 20 minutes, gently peel off the dried mask with your fingers and wash your face with water.

• Watermelon rind mask: Remove the red flesh from the watermelon. Cut off several pieces of the white rind (cut as thin as possible, around 1 mm) and apply them to the face, especially where acne and acne scars are present. The next day, large acne spots will usually be visibly smaller, and small ones will be obviously flattened, and scars will have faded significantly.

• Red bean paste detox mask: Wash 100 grams of red beans and boil until soft. Put the boiled red beans into the blender and purée them. Let them cool. Apply the red bean paste mask evenly to the face. Wash off with warm water after about 15 minutes. This mask has a good degreasing effect. Note: Be sure to boil the red beans until they are soft before use, to prevent rough particles from abrading the skin.

Chapter Seven
Getting Rid of Chloasma

Chloasma is pigmented skin that occurs on the face, and is a physiological change under the influence of various internal and external factors. According to TCM, it is caused by internal factors such as a deficiency of *qi* and blood, liver depression and *qi* stagnation, stagnation of *qi* and blood stasis, and dysfunction of meridians and viscera. Chloasma in women mostly occurs during pregnancy, postpartum, or middle age, and its formation is closely related to physical exhaustion, excessive psychological pressure, irregular menstruation, and constipation. It also occurs in a very small number of men.

Although there are differences in the location and depth of chloasma in each person, it mostly appears in the holographic acupoint areas of the facial meridians and organs, and its corresponding meridians and organs have clinical symptoms of deficiency of *qi* and blood and *qi* and blood stagnation of varying degrees of severity. Therefore, the health of the internal organs can be understood from the observation of chloasma's locations and forms. For the treatment of chloasma, in addition to unblocking the meridians of the parts on the face where *qi* and blood stagnation exist, it is more important to enhance and improve the condition of *qi* deficiency and blood stagnation of the relevant internal organs.

Note: Some acupoints involved in this book are distributed symmetrically on both sides of the body. When conducting facial *gua sha*, except for a few acupoints that require one-sided scraping, the rest are all symmetrical acupoints on both sides of the body by default.

Key Points of the Technique

1. Be sure to apply facial *gua sha* cream on the scraping area first. In the pre-treatment stage, the areas with pigmentations can be scraped once a day, 10 to 15 times each time, and changed to once every three days when the effect is obvious, 10 to 15 times each time.

2. First use the short-distance and slow-speed pushing and scraping method to scrape the chloasma. The scraping area should be slightly larger than the chloasma. Look carefully for positive reactions. Slight positive reactions are skin astringency, a fine, gravelly texture, and a bubbling sensation; obvious positive reactions are pain, nodules, and muscle tension and stiffness. The lighter the color of the chloasma, the smaller the area, and the smaller the positive reactant, the more slowly it needs to be scraped. The scraping speed should be controlled at 2 to 3 times within one calm breath.

3. The positive reactions can exist in the dermis, subcutaneous tissue, or even muscle according to the duration of the pigmentation, so the pressure should penetrate into the above layers of tissue. Look for the positive reactions, and do not press too hard. For a small positive reaction area, use the push-scraping method; for a large positive

reaction area, use the kneading and scraping method. The pressure should penetrate below the skin, above the muscle, or between the muscles at the positive reaction area.

4. In the early stage of scraping for chloasma removal, it is easy to find the positive reactions in the deeper layer, and the stagnant acupoints can be dredged faster, meaning that removal is faster and more obvious. In the later stage, the meridian stagnation acupoints become superficial, and the pressure should be gradually reduced. Flat-scraping or kneading and scraping will find or remove minor stasis acupoints in the superficial layers of the skin. Finding and eliminating the positive reactions under the chloasma is the key to success.

5. Chloasma is a reflection of *qi* deficiency and blood stasis inside the body, so it is necessary to scrape the relevant meridians at the same time, or the holographic acupoints corresponding to the viscera and organs. At the same time, it should be noted that the area scraped should not be too extensive each time, so as to avoid venting vital *qi*.

Chloasma on Both Sides of the Forehead and on Temples

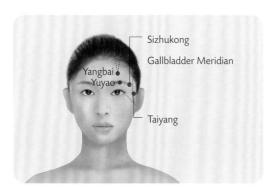

Chloasma on the forehead occurs mostly on the parts where the Gallbladder Meridian runs on both sides of the forehead. The chloasma here is caused by liver and gallbladder dysfunction, liver depression and *qi* stagnation, and often carries symptoms of weakened digestive function, insomnia, and excessive dreaming.

Facial Beauty *Gua Sha*

1. Clean the facial skin. After applying the facial *gua sha* cream, use the pushing and scraping method to scrape the forehead from the inside to the outside, focusing on the spots, as well as the Yangbai, Sizhukong, Yuyao, and Taiyang acupoints, scraping each acupoint 5 times. Look for positive reactions under the chloasma.

2. Use the flat-pressing and kneading method or the kneading and scraping method to scrape the positive reaction points under the chloasma. Scrape each part 10 times each time.

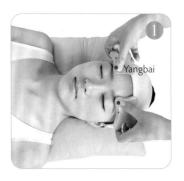
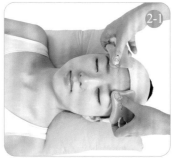
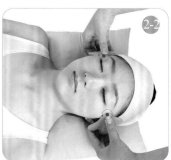

Consolidating *Gua Sha* on the Head and Neck

1. Use the surface-scraping to scrape the Gallbladder Meridian and the Triple Energizer meridian on the side of the head from front to back down.

    2. Use the sharp-edge scraping method to scrape the mid-frontal belt and the second lateral-frontal belt on the upper part of the chloasma.

    3. Use the single-angle scraping method to scrape the Fengchi acupoint on the neck, and use the surface-scraping method to scrape the Gallbladder Meridian area on the side of the neck.

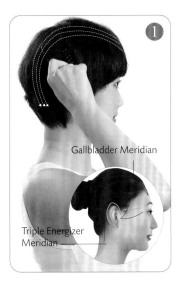
Gallbladder Meridian
Triple Energizer Meridian

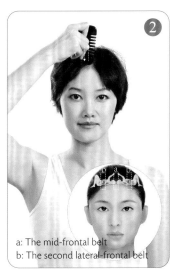
a: The mid-frontal belt
b: The second lateral-frontal belt

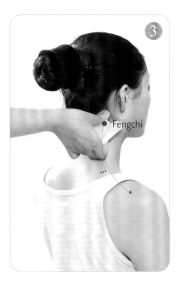
Fengchi

Whole-Body *Gua Sha* and Conditioning

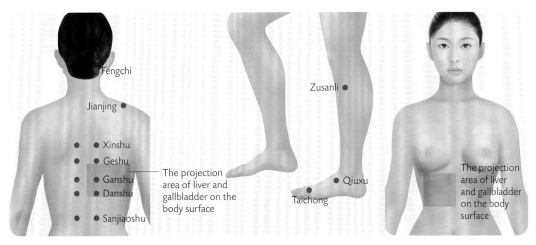

Fengchi
Jianjing
Xinshu
Geshu
Ganshu
Danshu
Sanjiaoshu
The projection area of liver and gallbladder on the body surface
Zusanli
Qiuxu
Taichong
The projection area of liver and gallbladder on the body surface

1. Use the surface-scraping method to scrape the Jianjing acupoint on the shoulder from the inside to the outside, and scrape the Xinshu acupoint from the top down to the Geshu, Ganshu, Danshu, and Sanjiaoshu acupoints.

    2. Use the flat-scraping method to scrape the projection area of liver and gallbladder on the right back and right flank from the inside to the outside.

3. Use the flat-pressing and kneading method to scrape the Zusanli acupoint on the lower limbs, use the flat-pressing and kneading method to scrape the Qiuxu acupoint, and use the vertical-pressing and kneading method to scrape the Taichong acupoint on the foot.

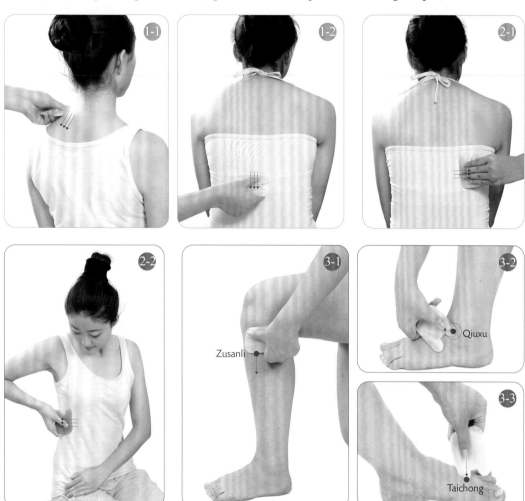

Expert Tip: A Good Mood Can Help Chloasma Fade

Soothing the liver and relieving depression, psychological adjustment is a good way to treat chloasma. People with chloasma are more or less related to sadness, depression, and emotional discomfort, especially the chloasma on both sides of the forehead. Scraping treatment can quickly promote blood circulation to remove blood stasis, clear blood vessels, but if you want to consolidate the effect of facial scraping and chloasma removal, you also need to scrape the meridian and holographic acupoint areas for soothing the liver and regulating *qi*. At the same time, you should pay attention to avoid overwork and overdraft of physical strength, and adjustment of emotions is especially necessary.

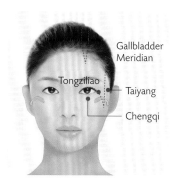

Gallbladder
Meridian

Tongziliao

Taiyang

Chengqi

Chloasma under the Outer Corner of the Eye

The appearance of chloasma under the outer corners of the eyes indicates that the shoulder joints are affected by wind-cold or the muscles of the neck and shoulders are strained. Neck and shoulder stiffness and soreness are often symptoms, so it is necessary to be alert to neck and shoulder diseases.

Facial Beauty *Gua Sha*

1. After cleansing the facial skin, apply facial *gua sha* cream, and use the pushing and scraping method to scrape the Tongziliao acupoint from the inside to the outer upper part.

2. Scrape the lower eyelid from the Chengqi acupoint, through the area corresponding to the neck, shoulders and upper limbs below the outer corner of the eye, to the Taiyang acupoints, with the pushing and scraping method, focusing on the stained area, and scrape each acupoint or acupoint area 5 times to find positive reactions.

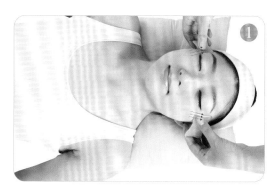

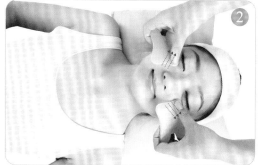

3. Focus on using the pushing and scraping method or the kneading and scraping method to scrape the stained parts and the positive reaction points under the Tongziliao acupoint, upper limb area, and the Taiyang acupoints, scrape each part 10 times.

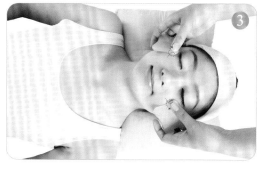

Consolidating *Gua Sha* **on the Head**

1. Use the surface-scraping method to scrape the Gallbladder Meridian and Triple Energizer Meridian on the side of the head from front to lower back.

2. Use the sharp-edge scraping method to scrape the mid-frontal belt, the second lateral-frontal belt, and the middle one-third area of the anterior and posterior oblique belt of the parieto-temporal region.

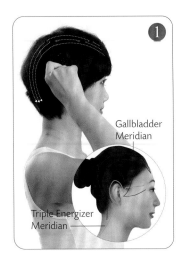

Gallbladder
Meridian

Triple Energizer
Meridian

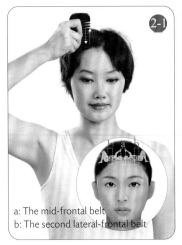

a: The mid-frontal belt
b: The second lateral-frontal belt

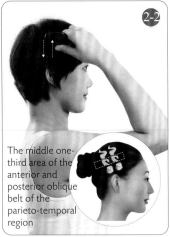

The middle one-third area of the anterior and posterior oblique belt of the parieto-temporal region

Whole-Body *Gua Sha* and Conditioning

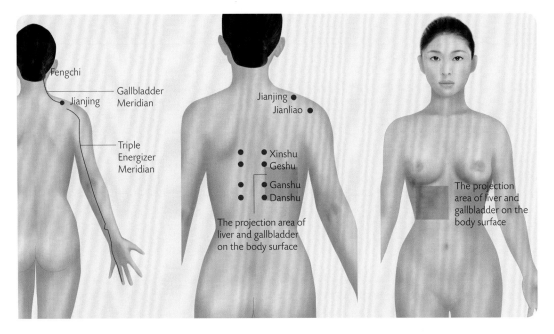

Fengchi

Jianjing

Gallbladder
Meridian

Triple
Energizer
Meridian

Jianjing
Jianliao

Xinshu
Geshu

Ganshu
Danshu

The projection area of
liver and gallbladder
on the body surface

The projection
area of liver and
gallbladder on the
body surface

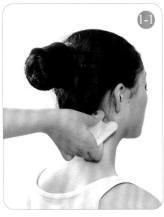

1. Scrape the Fengchi acupoint with the single-angle scraping method from top to bottom, scrape the Gallbladder Meridian on the neck with surface-scraping method. Scrape the Triple Energizer meridian and Waiguan acupoint on the upper limbs with the surface-scraping method from top to bottom. Vertically press and knead the Zhongzhu acupoint at the back of the hand.

2. Scrape the Jianjing and Jianliao acupoints. Use the surface-scraping method to scrape from the Xinshu acupoint to the Geshu, Ganshu, and Danshu acupoints from top to bottom.

3. Use the flat-scraping method to scrape the projection area of liver and gallbladder on the right back and right flank from the inside to the outside.

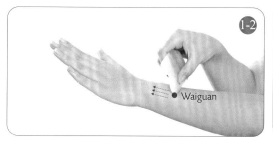

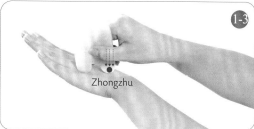

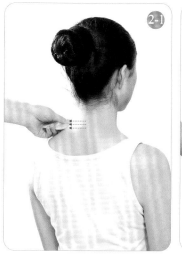

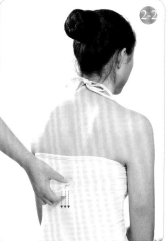

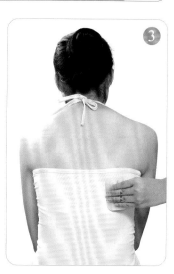

Expert Tip: Scraping the Neck and Shoulders and Keeping Warm Can Alleviate Chloasma

Muscle tension, weakened elasticity, lack of luster, and even chloasma below the outer corners of the eyes are manifestations of blood stagnation in the neck and shoulder area. Nowadays, there are more and more women with chloasma on this part of the face, which is not only related to excessive pressure in work and life and mental tension, but also to wearing strapless dresses and bending over the desk working for a long time in air-conditioned rooms. Women's shoulders are delicate and need to be kept warm, and when the neck and shoulders are attacked by wind and cold, it will lead to neck and shoulder pain and frozen shoulder. Even if the wind and cold are relatively mild, the local *qi* and blood will not run smoothly. In the alternating seasons of warm and cold, and when sleeping at night, make sure you keep your neck and shoulders warm. In addition, if you keep your upper limbs in a fixed position for a long time at work, do neck and shoulder exercises to relax. Doing the above can prevent chloasma in these areas. It can consolidate the effect of facial *gua sha* and chloasma removal for those who have already developed it.

Chloasma on the Bridge of the Nose

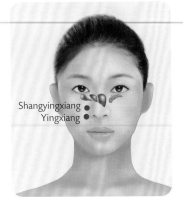

Shangyingxiang
Yingxiang

A greenish-yellow complexion with chloasma in the middle of the nose is mostly related to liver *qi* stagnation, emotional disorders or excessive mental stress, and decreased function of the spleen and stomach. It suggests liver dysfunction, and liver and gallbladder stagnation, and requires vigilance against liver and gallbladder disorders. Spots on the nose wings and root of the wings, which are the holographic acupoint areas of the stomach, can be signs of stomach and duodenal disorders.

Facial Beauty *Gua Sha*

1. Clean the facial skin. After applying facial *gua sha* cream, use the pushing and scraping method to scrape the liver area in the middle of the nose from top to bottom. Scrape the gallbladder and pancreas areas on both sides with the corner of the scraper, and scrape the Shangyingxiang and Yingxiang acupoints from the inside to the outside and above, focusing on the chloasma area. Look for positive reactions, and scrape each acupoint area 5 times.

2. Scrape the positive reaction points on the pigmented area with the pushing and scraping method 10 times, and use the flat-pressing and kneading method to scrape the Shangyingxiang and Yingxiang acupoints 10 times.

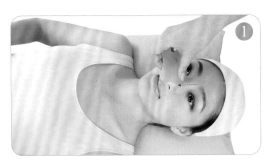

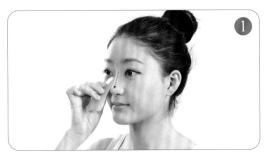

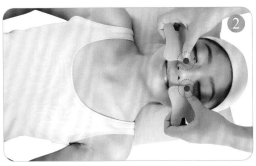

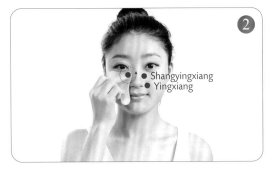

Shangyingxiang
Yingxiang

Consolidating *Gua Sha* on the Head and Neck

1. Use the sharp-edge scraping method to scrape the mid-frontal belt, the second lateral-frontal belt, and the middle one-third area of the frontal belt of the head top.

2. First use the surface-scraping method to scrape the Governor Vessel area of the

1st to 5th cervical vertebra from top to bottom, and then use the dual-angle scraping method to scrape the Bladder Meridian area on both sides.

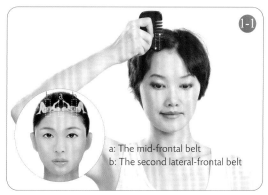
a: The mid-frontal belt
b: The second lateral-frontal belt

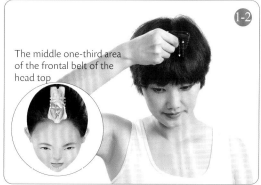
The middle one-third area of the frontal belt of the head top

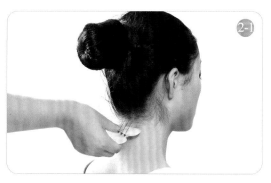

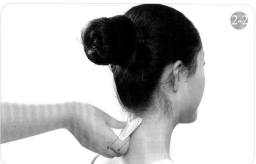

Whole-Body *Gua Sha* and Conditioning

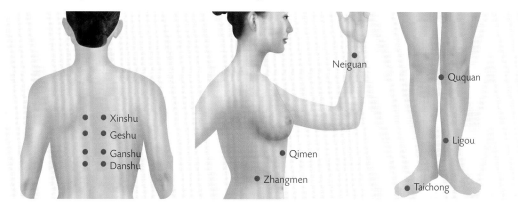

1. Use the surface-scraping method to scrape the Xinshu, Geshu, Ganshu, and Danshu acupoints from top to bottom.

2. Use the surface-scraping method to scrape the Qimen and Zhangmen acupoints from top to bottom separately.

3. Use the surface-scraping method to scrape the Neiguan acupoints on the upper limbs, and the Ququan and Ligou acupoints on the lower limbs from top to bottom. Press and knead the Taichong acupoint on the foot with the vertical-pressing and kneading method.

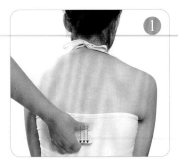

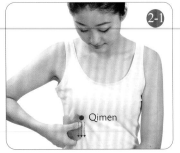

Qimen

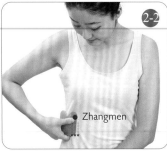

Zhangmen

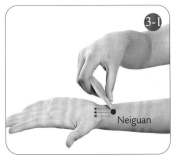

Neiguan

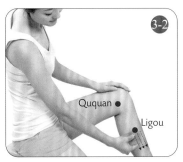

Ququan

Ligou

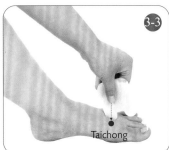

Taichong

Expert Tip: The Color of Your Nose Can Indicate Your Mood and Health

The color of the middle of the nose can reveal a person's mood and the health of their liver. Anyone who is chronically stressed, depressed or has decreased liver function will have a darker color in the middle of the nose.

Unpleasant emotions will eventually lead to a stagnation of *qi* in the body, and a constitution prone to blood stasis is prone to developing pigmented spots on the face. In addition, hyperplasia of the mammary glands is a common and frequently-occurring condition in women, and is closely related to liver depression and *qi* stagnation. Holographic scraping and scraping the corresponding area of the breast on the back has a significant effect on the treatment of breast hyperplasia.

Divide the area of the back corresponding to the mammary glands into four areas with a cross. Apply scraping oil, and scrape from top to bottom in order, focusing on finding the pain points and nodules in the corresponding area.

Scraping the Ganshu, Danshu, and Gaohuang acupoints on the Bladder Meridian, the Jianjing acupoint on the Gallbladder Meridian, and the Tianzong acupoint on the Small Intestine Meridian can soothe the liver and relieve depression, promote blood circulation and disperse nodules, consolidating the effect.

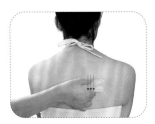

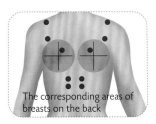

The corresponding areas of breasts on the back

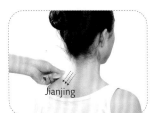

Jianjing

Chloasma on the Cheek Areas

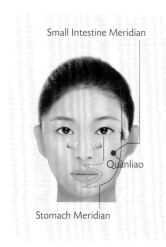

Small Intestine Meridian

Quanliao

Stomach Meridian

The two zygomatic areas are the holographic acupoint area of the small intestine and the part where the Small Intestine Meridian and Stomach Meridian run. Chloasma in the center of the two zygomas is often accompanied by shortness of breath, fatigue, palpitations, chest tightness, decreased digestive function, and even loss of appetite, abdominal distension, and diarrhea. It is a manifestation of a weakened digestive system and heart function.

From the two zygomatic areas to the front of the ear is the holographic acupoint area of the kidneys, and there are many meridians running through it. Chloasma in this part indicates a deficiency of kidney *qi*, stagnation of *qi* circulation in the triple energizer, and disordered lipid metabolism.

Facial Beauty *Gua Sha*

1. Clean the facial skin, apply facial *gua sha* cream, and then use the pushing and scraping method first to scrape the Quanliao acupoint from the bottom upwards, and then scrape the small intestine area and the chloasma area on the cheeks from the inside outwards and upwards. Look for the positive reaction points, and push and scrape 5 times for each acupoint area. Scrape 10 times on the positive reaction areas found with pushing and scraping method or kneading and scraping method.

2. Use the pushing and scraping method to scrape the kidney area in front of the ear from the inside to the outside and upwards, focusing on the chloasma area. Look for positive reaction points, and scrape 5 times each. Then use the pushing and scraping method or kneading and scraping method to scrape 10 times at the positive reaction points.

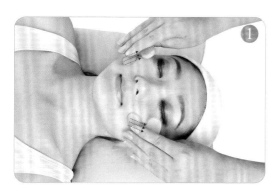

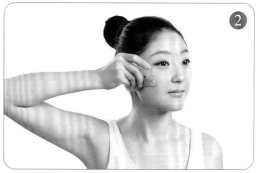

Consolidating *Gua Sha* on the Head, Hands, and Feet

1. Use the sharp-edge scraping method to scrape the first lateral-frontal belt and third lateral-frontal belt on the head.

2. Scrape the thenar, hypothenar areas and the heart, kidney areas in the sole with the pushing and scraping method.

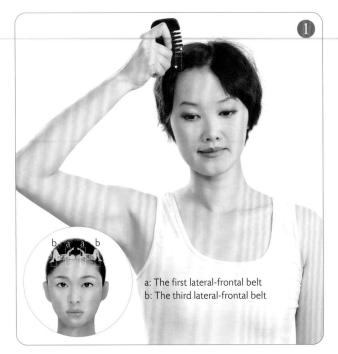

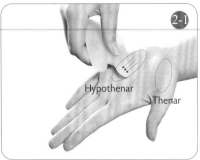

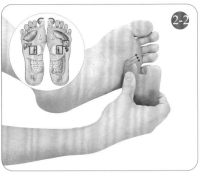

a: The first lateral-frontal belt
b: The third lateral-frontal belt

Hypothenar   Thenar

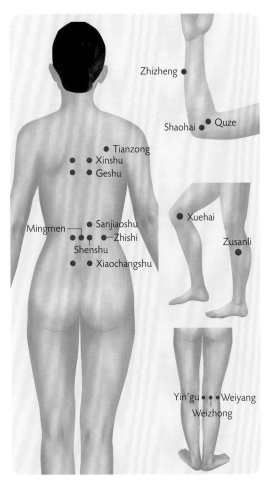

Zhizheng

Shaohai ● ● Quze

● Tianzong
● ● Xinshu
● ● Geshu

Mingmen   ● Sanjiaoshu
● ● ● —Zhishi
Shenshu
● Xiaochangshu

● Xuehai

Zusanli

Yin'gu ● ● Weiyang
Weizhong

Whole-Body *Gua Sha* and Conditioning

For chloasma on the cheekbones: 1. Use the surface-scraping method to scrape the Xinshu, Geshu, Xiaochangshu, and Tianzong acupoints on the back from top to bottom. 2. Use the surface-scraping method to scrape the Xiaohai and Zhizheng acupoints on the upper limbs from top to bottom. Use the clapping method to pat the Quze and Shaohai acupoints in the elbow pit. Scrape the Zusanli and Xuehai acupoints on the lower limbs from top to bottom.

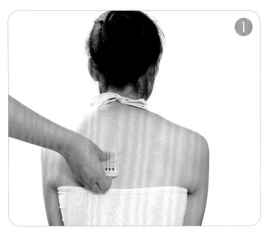

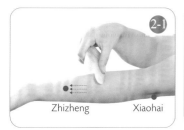
Zhizheng   Xiaohai

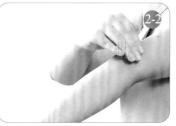

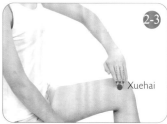
Xuehai

For chloasma from the cheeks to the kidney area in front of the ear: 1. Use the surface-scraping method to scrape the Mingmen, Sanjiaoshu, Shenshu, and Zhishi acupoints on the back from top to bottom. 2. Use the clapping method to pat the Weizhong, Weiyang, and Yin'gu acupoints on the lower limbs.

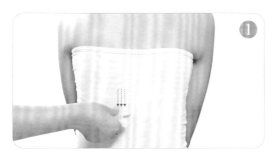

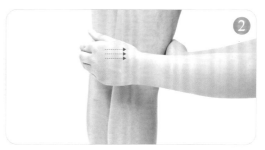

Expert Tip: Unique Features of Scraping for Chloasma Removal and Whitening

The formation of chloasma is related to internal issues such as genetic factors, female hormone imbalance, pregnancy, childbirth, menstruation, internal organ problems, mental stress, and skin aging. It is also related to external factors such as sun exposure or long-term use of cosmetics containing fragrances, lead, and mercury. Ultraviolet rays are the number one cause of chloasma. Excessive exposure to the sun without proper protection can lead to sun spots and spot deepening.

Pigmentation is often in the base layer of the skin. Many cosmetic and anti-freckle products only act on the epidermal tissue, and it is difficult for the active ingredients to interact with the melanin in the base layer. *Gua Sha* works from the upper and lower aspects of the skin, promoting the metabolism of the skin and accelerating the decomposition of melanin. It also promotes the circulation of meridians, improves the microcirculation of skin tissues, and allows the metabolic waste that stagnates in the blood vessels and darkens the skin tone to be carried away from the blood in the veins beneath the skin. After scraping away blood stasis and dredging the meridians, fresh, clean, nutrient-rich blood is supplied continuously to the skin cells, and the unimpeded blood vessels can continue to take away waste products. This is the principle of facial *gua sha* for chloasma removal and whitening .

Chloasma on the Upper Lip

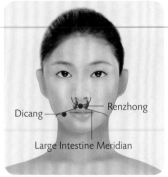

Chloasma on the skin of the upper lip is a sign of insufficient kidney *qi* and large intestine deficiency-cold. It is often accompanied by symptoms of constipation and irregular menstruation, and can be a sign of uterine and ovarian issues.

Facial Beauty *Gua Sha*

1. Clean the facial skin, apply facial *gua sha* cream, and scrape the Renzhong acupoint on the upper lip with the pushing and scraping method. Then push and scrape from the Renzhong acupoint to the Dicang acupoint, focusing on finding and scraping the positive reaction areas under the chloasma. Scrape each area 5 times.

2. Use the pushing and scraping method or flat-pressing and kneading method to scrape the positive reaction areas at the chloasma on the upper lip, and scrape 10 times.

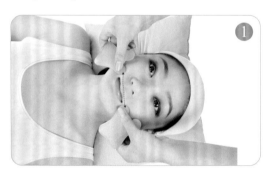

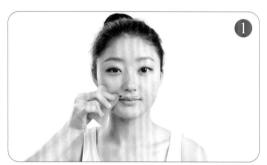

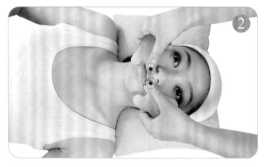

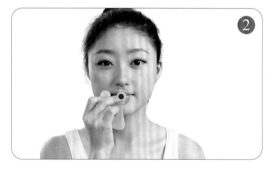

Consolidating *Gua Sha* on the Head, Hands, and Feet

1. Use the sharp-edge scraping method to scrape the mid-frontal belt, the second lateral-frontal belt, and the middle one-third area of the frontal belt of the head top, and the rear one-third area of the frontal belt of the head top.

2. Scrape the kidney area and uterus area in the palm with the pushing and scraping method.

3. Scrape the gonad area in the sole and at the inner and outer sides of the heel with the pushing and scraping method.

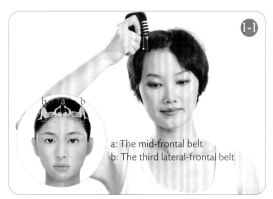

a: The mid-frontal belt
b: The third lateral-frontal belt

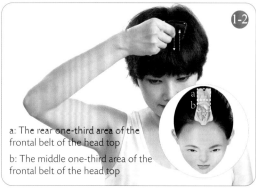

a: The rear one-third area of the frontal belt of the head top

b: The middle one-third area of the frontal belt of the head top

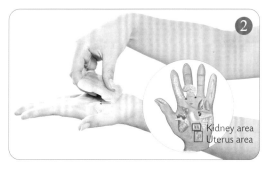

☐ Kidney area
☐ Uterus area

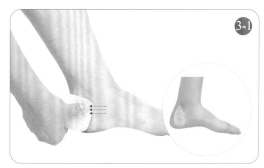

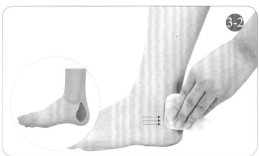

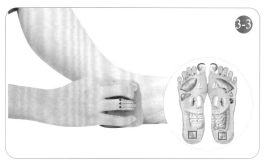

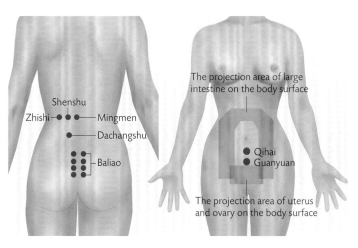

Shenshu
Zhishi — Mingmen
Dachangshu
Baliao

The projection area of large intestine on the body surface

Qihai
Guanyuan

The projection area of uterus and ovary on the body surface

Whole-Body *Gua Sha* and Conditioning

1. Use the surface-scraping method to scrape the Mingmen, Shenshu, Zhishi, Dachangshu, and Baliao acupoints on the back from top to bottom.

2. Use the surface-scraping method to scrape the projection area of large intestine, uterus, and ovary on the body surface from top to bottom, focusing on the Qihai acupoint to the Guanyuan acupoint.

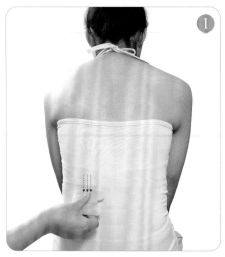

①

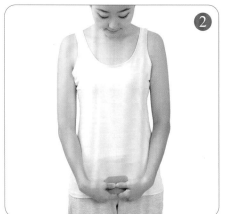

②

Expert Tip: Regular Menstruation Helps Eliminate Chloasma

Women with chloasma often experience irregular menstruation, which is caused by an underlying ovulatory disorder. The status of ovulation is related to the gonadal axis including the ovaries, hypothalamus, and pituitary gland. Problems with any part of this axis, especially the hypothalamus and pituitary gland, can lead to irregular menstruation and amenorrhea. Irregular menstruation can be a sign of dysfunction of the gonadal axis as well as a sign of systemic dysfunction.

If there are changes in your menstrual period such as in the volume and color, or amenorrhea, dysmenorrhea, or persistent menstruation, it is important to consult a doctor immediately. In a sense, irregular menstruation is a harbinger of disease and difficulty conceiving.

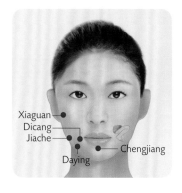

Xiaguan
Dicang
Jiache
Daying
Chengjiang

Chloasma on the Lateral Sides of the Lower Jaw

Chloasma on the lateral side of the lower jaw is a sign of poor blood circulation in the lower limbs and a deficiency of spleen and kidney *qi*. It is often characterized by soreness of the lower limbs, soreness and weakness in the waist and knees, cold hands and feet, and weakened digestion function.

Facial Beauty *Gua Sha*

1. Clean the facial skin. After applying facial *gua sha* cream, scrape the Chengjiang acupoint with the pushing and scraping method, focusing on the pigmented area of the lower jaw. Look for positive reaction points, and scrape 5 times each. Press and knead the positive reaction points under the chloasma with the flat-pressing and kneading method, and scrape 10 times.

2. Use the pushing and scraping method to scrape the Dicang, Daying, lower limb area, Jiache, and Xiaguan acupoints from the inside to the outside and upwards, focusing on the pigmented area. Look for positive reaction points, and scrape each point 5 times. Use the pushing and scraping method or kneading and scraping method to scrape the positive reaction points in the facial lower limb area and on the chloasma, and scrape 10 times.

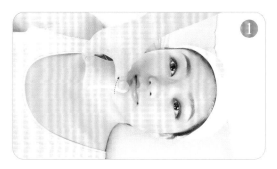 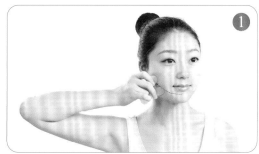

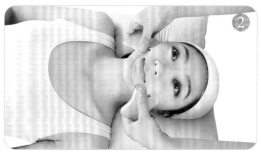 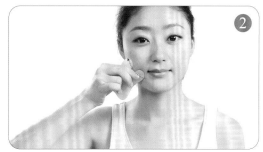

Consolidating *Gua Sha* on the Head

Scrape the middle one-third area of the frontal belt of the head top, and the rear one-third area of the frontal belt of the head top, and the middle one-third area of the anterior and posterior oblique belt of the parieto-temporal region with the sharp-edge scraping method.

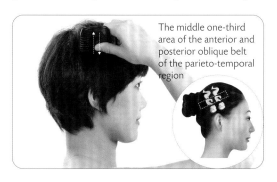 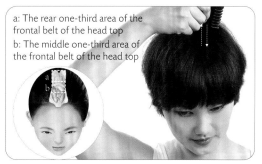

Whole-Body *Gua Sha* and Conditioning

1. Use the surface-scraping method to scrape the Mingmen, Pishu, Weishu, Shenshu, and Zhishi acupoints on the back from top to bottom.

2. Use the clapping method to tap the Weizhong, Weiyang, and Yin'gu acupoints on the lower limbs. Use the surface-scraping method to scrape the Xiyangguan, Yanglingquan, and Zusanli acupoints on the lower limbs from top to bottom.

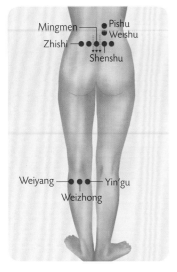

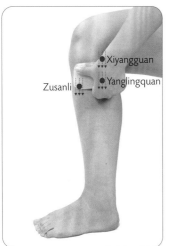

The treatment of chloasma should not only focus on tonifying *qi* and blood, but also promoting blood circulation to remove blood stasis. *Gua Sha* improves the microcirculation of the skin, fills the skin with *qi* and blood, removes chloasma and whitens the skin, and at the same time promotes blood circulation to remove blood stasis on the connected meridians and corresponding viscera and organs. It also clears the meridians, promotes blood circulation to remove blood stasis, and tonifies *qi* and blood, because smooth meridians will bring rich nutrients to skin cells, viscera, and organs. This is how *gua sha* "tonifies by dredging," completing "dredging" and "tonifying" at the same time.

To treat chloasma with *gua sha* therapy, you must master the "degree" of scraping. This is because the causes of chloasma are insufficient *qi* and blood, and blood stasis due to deficiency, so each site should not be scraped too many times, nor for too long time in order to avoid excessive opening of the pores, which can let out vital *qi*.

Diet Therapy and Skin Care

Eat more foods rich in vitamins C and E, such as Chinese cabbage, winter melon, white radish, lemons, apples, tomatoes, peanuts, lettuce, lean meat, and egg yolk. Eat less pigmented foods such as soy sauce and pickles. Avoid tobacco, alcohol, and coffee.

Food Therapy Recipes
• Yam porridge with wolfberries: Wash 100 grams of japonica rice, soak in cold water for 1 hour, remove and drain. Take 50 grams of fresh yam, and peel, scrape, and wash. Cut into small cubes for later use. Soak 15 grams of wolfberries in warm water and set aside. Add 1500 milliliter of cold water to a pot, add japonica rice, yam, and wolfberries, bring to a boil over a high heat, then turn to a low heat and simmer until very soft. Add 15 grams of sugar and 10 grams of honey to serve. This porridge nourishes the blood and skin, and eliminates chloasma.

• Fruit soup: Take 1 pear, 1 apple, 1 banana, 1 pineapple, 1 kiwi, and 4 strawberries, and wash and dice for later use. Add an appropriate amount of water to a pot, put in the diced fruit, bring to a boil over a high heat, and then turn to a low heat to simmer. When the fruit is boiled, add 15 grams of white sugar, and finally pour in 20 grams of water starch, pushing it into the fruit with a spoon as you pour. Boil it, put it into a soup basin, let it cool, add 10 grams of honey, and serve. This porridge relieves summer heat and irritation, whitens the skin, and removes chloasma.

• Coix seed and lotus seed porridge: Wash 150 grams of coix seeds, soak in cold water for 3 hours, remove and drain. Take 50 grams of lotus seeds, remove the pits and wash with cold water. Wash and remove the pits of 5 red dates. Add 1000 milliliter of cold water to the pot, add the coix seeds, bring to the boil over a high heat, then add lotus seeds and red dates, and simmer until cooked through. Finally, add 15 grams of rock sugar, simmer until it becomes porridge, and then eat. This porridge whitens and moisturizes the skin, and can eliminate freckles, age spots, and butterfly stains.

• Loquat and red date porridge: Rinse 6 loquats, peel off the skin, and remove the core. Wash 100 grams of japonica rice, soak in cold water for 1 hour, remove and drain. Add 1000 milliliter of cold water to the pot, add japonica rice and red dates, bring to a boil over high heat, add the loquats, switch to a low heat and cook into porridge. Add sugar to taste and serve. This porridge nourishes the lungs and skin, removes chloasma, and strengthens the stomach.

• Orange and hawthorn congee: Peel 2 oranges, tear off the veins, separate the segments, remove the seeds with a tooth pick, and cut into small triangles. Wash 30 grams of hawthorn berries and cut each into two halves, removing the seeds. Wash 100 grams of japonica rice, soak in cold water for 1 hour, remove and drain. Add 1500 milliliter of cold water to the pot, add japonica rice, orange pieces, and hawthorn pieces, bring to the boil over a high heat, switch to a low heat and cook into porridge. Add 10 grams of sugar and serve. This porridge can nourish and protect the skin, and remove dark spots.

Homemade Chloasma Removal Masks

• Apple mask: Put 4 pieces of apple into a food blender and mash into juice. Add honey and mix well. Refrigerate for about 10 minutes. Pat the mixture over the entire face with your hands until it feels slightly sticky. Rinse it off with water after about 30 minutes. This mask is suitable for normal skin.

• Banana mask: Peel bananas and mash them into a paste. Apply to the face and cover. Peel off the mask after 15 to 20 minutes and wash off. Long-term use can make the facial skin tender and refreshed, and is suitable for dry or sensitive skin.

• Tomato, lemon and oatmeal mask: Combine 1 cup tomato juice, 1 tbsp lemon juice, and 1 tbsp instant oatmeal. Stir well and apply to the entire face, concentrating on areas of the cheeks, forehead, and chin with more spots. If necessary, add a little more oatmeal to the mixture to make it thicker. Leave the mask on for about 10 minutes, then wipe it off with a damp, hot towel. This mask can remove chloasma and nourish the skin.

CHAPTER EIGHT

Tightening Pores and Reducing Eye Bags

There are two main reasons for rough skin and enlarged pores. The first is seborrhea. From puberty, some people's sebaceous glands are over-active, and the oil secretions of the skin and hair are too much, resulting in enlarged pores. The second is photoaging, i.e., symptoms of premature skin aging due to excessive sun exposure. In addition to enlarged pores and rough skin, wrinkles or pigmented spots may also appear.

Scraping the facial skin can activate the metabolic function of skin cells, enhance their self-cleaning function, and accelerate the discharge of metabolic waste clogged in pores. It can also unblock and clean pores, improve the blood circulation of the face, and promote the shrinkage function of skin pores to shrink pores.

Note: Some acupoints involved in this book are distributed symmetrically on both sides of the body. When conducting facial *gua sha*, except for a few acupoints that require one-sided scraping, the rest are all symmetrical acupoints on both sides of the body by default.

Key Points for Pores Tightening

1. Be sure to apply facial *gua sha* cream on the treatment area first, and use flat-pressing and kneading method and flat-scraping method. The pressure should penetrate the soft tissue under the skin and above the muscles.

2. The speed of scraping should be slow, controlled to scrape 2 to 3 times within one calm breath. Do not press too hard or scrape too fast.

3. After facial *gua sha*, cleanse the skin and then apply toner and moisturizer. People with excessive oil secretion should clean their skin thoroughly to avoid residual facial *gua sha* cream from clogging the pores.

4. Do not scrape areas affected by acne or rosacea. Scraping should only be performed after the inflammation is eliminated and the local skin color returns to normal.

Gua Sha Steps for Large Pores on the Forehead and Nose

The lungs govern the skin and hair. The middle and lower part of the forehead is the holographic acupoint area of the lungs, and is also the area where the Governor Vessel and the Bladder Meridian run. This part is most likely to have enlarged pores. Merely enlarged pores are mostly manifestations of a deficiency of lung *qi*. Enlarged pores combined with a smaller shape, slight sunkenness, and a lack of luster are external symptoms of lung and kidney deficiency, and there will also be shortness of breath, fatigue, and weakness.

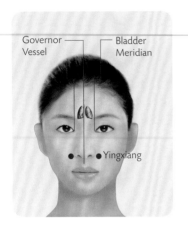

Governor
Vessel

Bladder
Meridian

Yingxiang

The nose is the lung orifice, and also the holographic acupoint area of the spleen and stomach. The Yingxiang acupoint next to the nose is the acupoint of the Large Intestine Meridian. Enlarged pores on the nose are a manifestation of spleen and lung *qi* deficiency. At first, enlarged pores often appear at the Yingxiang acupoint next to the nose, and then gradually appear at the tip of the nose, often with symptoms of shortness of breath, loss of appetite, and constipation. If the pores are enlarged and the skin is red, it means that the lung *qi* deficiency is accompanied by deficiency-fire and internal heat.

Facial Beauty *Gua Sha*

1. After cleansing the skin, apply facial *gua sha* cream, scrape from top to bottom according to the sequence of the different *gua sha* methods for different parts of the face, from the forehead, around the eyes, the cheeks, around the mouth, nose, and to the jaw. Use the skin-lubricating and wrinkle-removing method to scrape each part 5 times. On this basis, focus on scraping the areas with enlarged pores with the flat-scraping method, the flat-pressing and kneading method. Scrape every 3 to 5 days to make the pores smaller and the skin delicate and smooth.

2. Use the pushing and scraping method to find and locate positive reaction points in the lung area of the forehead, the nosal area, and the cheeks under the Yingxiang acupoints, and scrape each acupoint area 5 times.

3. Use the flat-pressing and kneading method to press and knead the forehead, nose, and Yingxiang acupoints with enlarged pores, scraping 10 times for each area, until the skin is slightly warm and flushed.

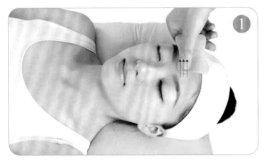

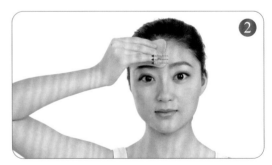

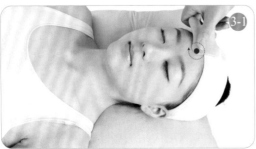

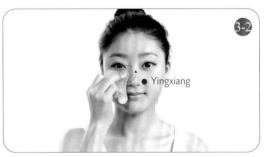

Yingxiang

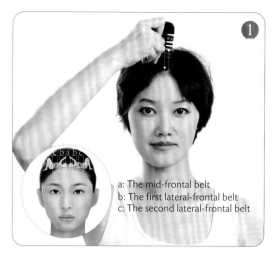

a: The mid-frontal belt
b: The first lateral-frontal belt
c: The second lateral-frontal belt

Consolidating *Gua Sha* on the Head, Hands and Feet

1. Scrape the mid-frontal belt, the first lateral-frontal belt and second lateral-frontal belt on both sides of the head with the sharp-edge scraping method.

2. Use the groove of the scraper to scrape the thumb and index finger in sequence, and then use the side of the scraper to scrape the lung area and large intestine area in the hands and feet with the flat-scraping method.

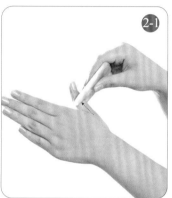

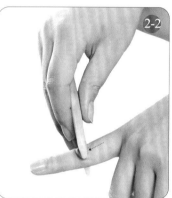

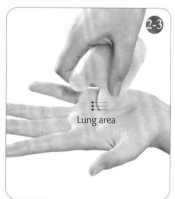

Lung area

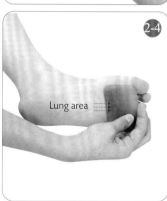

Lung area

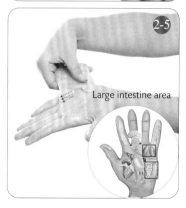

Large intestine area

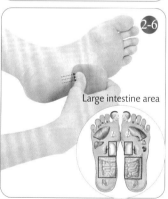

Large intestine area

Whole-Body *Gua Sha* and Conditioning

1. Use the surface-scraping method to scrape the Feishu, Pishu, Weishu, Sanjiaoshu, and Dachangshu acupoints on both sides of the back from top to bottom.

2. Use the single-angle scraping method to scrape the Danzhong and Zhongfu acupoints from top to bottom. Use the surface-scraping method to scrape the Dabao acupoint from top to bottom.

3. Scrape the Lung Meridian, the Large Intestine Meridian on the arm, and the Triple Energizer Meridian in the outer middle region of the arm with a scraper through

the clothes. Focus on scraping the bilateral Lieque, Taiyuan, and Quchi acupoints, and pressing and kneading the Hegu acupoints. Scrape the Zusanli acupoints on both sides of the lower limbs through clothes, or flat-press and knead the Zusanli acupoints.

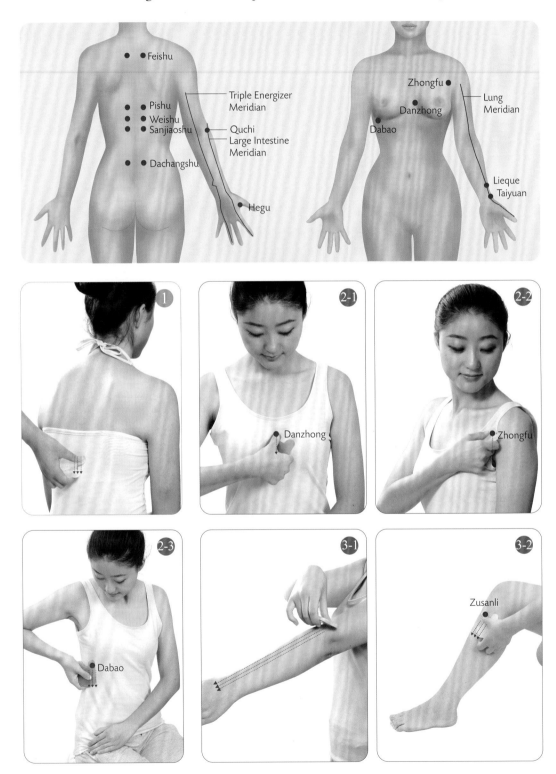

Diet Therapy and Skin Care for Tightening Pores

• To reduce the skin's oil secretion and make the pores smaller, eat leeks, spinach, radishes, winter melon, loofah, celery, cucumber, tomatoes, watermelon, pears, and bananas, and drink green tea and take vitamin C supplements.

• Keep stools smooth by regularly consuming crude fiber or intestinal detoxification foodstuffs, especially coarse grains and tubers.

• Drink plenty of water to clean your skin. Avoid spicy foods, alcohol, and stimulating food, as well as sweets and food containing too much oil.

Food Therapy Recipes

• Radish porridge: 1 large white radish, 50 grams of japonica rice. First cut the radish into small cubes, and then cook it with japonica rice into porridge. Eat it to cleanse your face and make the skin delicate.

• Sesame porridge: Stir-fry sesame seeds, add a small amount of fine salt, sprinkle on porridge and mix well; put 25 grams of sesame seeds in each bowl of porridge. Eat two bowls a day to moisturize your skin.

• Red date porridge: Take 10 red dates, cook them with 50 grams of japonica rice to make porridge, and eat it before going to bed to strengthen the spleen and *qi*, nourish blood, and moisturize your skin.

• Lily porridge: Take 30 grams of fresh lily (or 15 grams of dried lily), 50 grams of japonica rice, and an appropriate amount of rock sugar. Cook the japonica rice porridge first; add the lily when the porridge is 80% cooked, and then cook until it is ready. Eat it every night with a little rock sugar to nourish the lungs and *yin*, and moisturize your skin.

Homemade Face Mask
Honey and milk mask: 50 milliliters of milk, 5 grams of honey, 1 egg white, 5 milliliters of peppermint oil, 5 milliliters of lemon juice. First mix the milk, honey, and egg white together, then add a small amount of peppermint oil and lemon juice and stir quickly; apply to the face, leave for 15 to 20 minutes, and then wash off. Egg whites and lemons are the best partners for firming the skin, while honey and milk can moisturize and smooth it.

Key Points for Reducing Eye Bags

Because the eyelid skin is very thin and the subcutaneous tissue is loose, sagging and edema are prone to occur. Heredity is an important factor, and it becomes more pronounced with age. In addition, lipid metabolism disorders, hyperlipidemia, diseases of the kidneys, spleen, and stomach, pregnancy, lack of sleep or fatigue can cause eye skin to sag, and an accumulation of body fluids or fat can form bags under the eyes.

TCM holds that the formation of bags under the eyes is related to a disorder of *qi* and blood in the meridians and viscera: the lower eyelid is the holographic point corresponding to the small intestine, and it is also the starting point of the Stomach Meridian; the inner corner of the eye is the starting point of the Bladder Meridian, and the outer corner of the eye is the starting point of the Gallbladder Meridian; the lower eye socket is where the Liver Meridian runs. On the surface, the formation of bags under the eyes is related to the Stomach Meridian, Gallbladder Meridian, and Bladder Meridian, but in essence it is the result of a decline and imbalance of the spleen, liver, and kidneys. Scraping to reduce bags under the eyes should go as follows:

• Apply facial *gua sha* cream on the treatment area first, and prevent it from getting into the eyes during the scraping process.

• To remove minor bags under the eyes or prevent them from forming, use flat-pressing and kneading method and pushing and scraping method. The speed should be slow, controlled to scrape 1 to 2 times within one calm breath.

• For obvious and loose eye bags, when scraping the lower eyelid with the pushing and scraping method, the advancing distance each time should be short, between 1 and 2 millimeters. Between each scraping motion, the scraper should be lifted off the skin to avoid continuous pulling and tugging of the skin, causing the eyelid skin to loosen.

• The pressure of scraping and pressing should penetrate the soft tissue under the skin and above the muscles. Look for positive reactions such as gravel and nodules in the eye bags of the lower eyelids. For soft nodules formed by fatty tissue, scrape with the flat-pressing and kneading method.

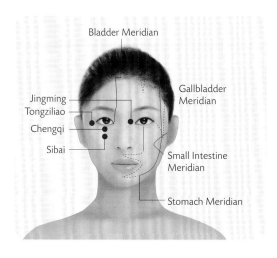

Bladder Meridian

Gallbladder Meridian

Jingming
Tongziliao

Chengqi

Sibai

Small Intestine Meridian

Stomach Meridian

Gua Sha Steps for Reducing Eye Bags

Premature bags under the eyes are a manifestation of spleen and stomach *qi* deficiency. Loose eye bags, sagging, and obvious wrinkles are manifestations of spleen deficiency, with symptoms such as loss of appetite, weakened digestive function, abdominal distension, diarrhea, or inability to defecate. People with full and swollen eye bags often have damp heat in the spleen and stomach, with a strong appetite, which is a sign of disordered fat metabolism and increased blood lipids. Those with full and bulging bags under the eyes long term should be alert to arteriosclerosis, and should seek medical attention for early detection and treatment.

Facial Beauty *Gua Sha*

1. After cleansing the skin, apply facial *gua sha* cream. Press and knead the Jingming acupoint with the vertical-pressing and kneading method, then scrape the Chengqi, Sibai and Tongziliao acupoints with the pushing and scraping method. Focus on looking for the gravel nodule form of positive reactions in the bags under the eyes. Scrape each part 5 times.

2. Press and knead the positive reaction area of the eye bags, and scrape each part 5 times with the flat-pressing and kneading method.

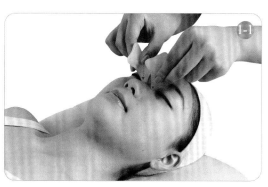

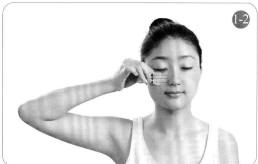

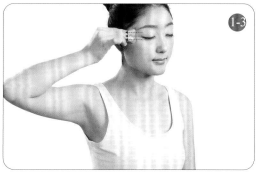

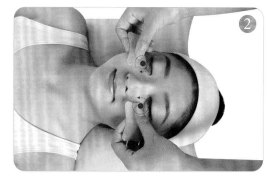

Consolidating *Gua Sha* on the Head, Hands and Feet

1. Use the sharp-edge scraping method to scrape the second lateral-frontal belt and the third lateral-frontal belt on both sides of the head.

2. Scrape the thenar and hypothenar, and the stomach, liver, and kidney areas of the feet with the surface-scraping method.

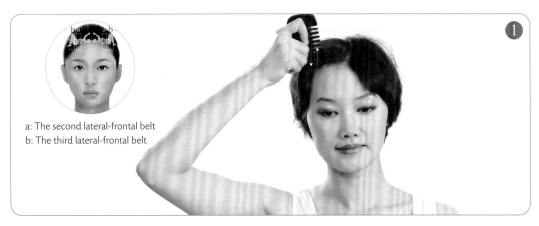

a: The second lateral-frontal belt
b: The third lateral-frontal belt

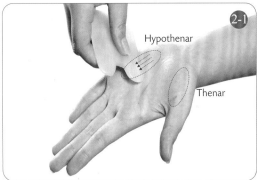

Hypothenar

Thenar

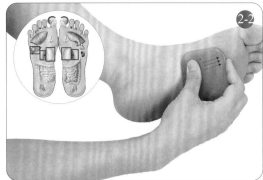

Whole-Body *Gua Sha* and Conditioning

For those with loose and drooping bags under the eyes: 1. Scrape the corresponding area of spleen and stomach on the spine. ① Use the facial scraping method to scrape the Governor Vessel of the 8th to 12th thoracic vertebrae from top to bottom. ② Use the dual-angle scraping method to scrape the Jiaji acupoints from top to bottom on both sides of the same horizontal section of the Governor Vessel. ③ Use the surface-scraping method to scrape the 3-cun wide area on both sides of the Governor Vessel from top to bottom. Focus on scraping the Pishu and Weishu acupoints.

2. Use the flat-scraping method from inside to outside along the ribs to scrape the surface projection area of spleen and pancreas on the left chest rib region and on the left back, and scrape the Zhongwan and Qihai acupoints on the abdomen from top to bottom.

3. Use the surface-scraping method from top to bottom or press and knead the Waiguan acupoints on the upper limbs with the flat-pressing and kneading method, and the Zusanli, Yinlingquan, Sanyinjiao and Gongsun acupoints on the lower limbs.

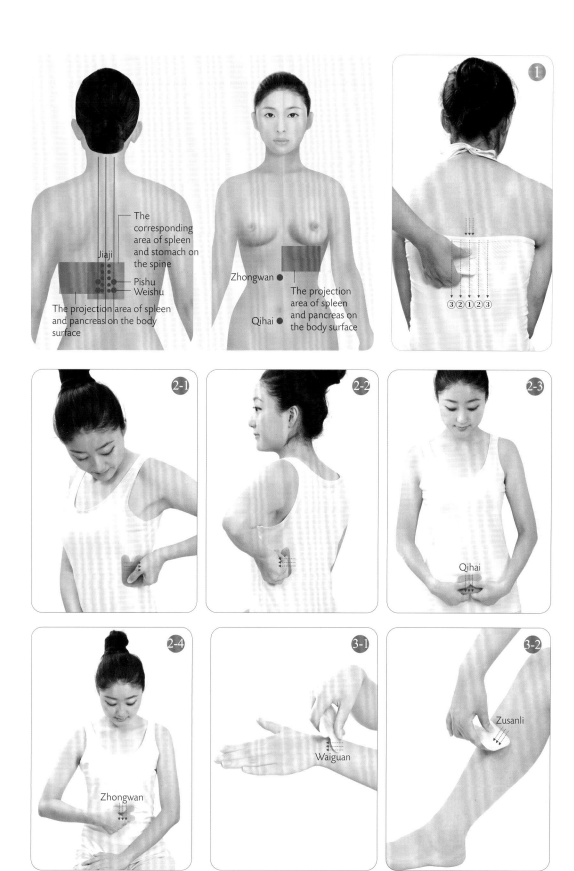

The
corresponding
area of spleen
and stomach on
the spine

Jiaji

Pishu
Weishu

The projection area of spleen
and pancreas on the body
surface

Zhongwan ●

The projection
area of spleen
and pancreas on
the body surface

Qihai ●

① ③②①②③

② 2-1

② 2-2

② 2-3

Qihai

② 2-4

Zhongwan

③ 3-1

Waiguan

③ 3-2

Zusanli

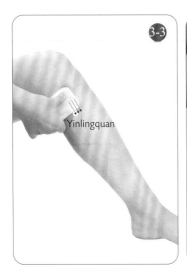

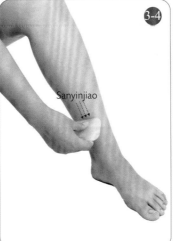

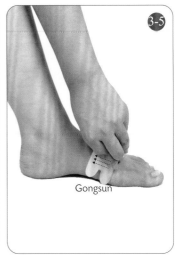

3-3 Yinlingquan

3-4 Sanyinjiao

3-5 Gongsun

For those with full and bulging eye bags: 1. Scrape the corresponding area of liver the gallbladder on the spine. ① Use the surface-scraping method to scrape the Governor Vessel between the 5th to 10th thoracic vertebrae from top to bottom. ② Use the dual-angle scraping method to scrape the Jiaji acupoints at the same level. ③ Finally, use the surface-scraping method to scrape a 3-cun wide area on both sides. Focus on scraping the Ganshu, Danshu, Pishu, Weishu, and Shenshu acupoints on both sides.

2. Use the flat-scraping method to scrape the projection area of liver and gallbladder on the right chest rib region and on the right back from the inside to the outside along the direction of the ribs.

3. Use the surface-scraping method to scrape the Fenglong and Shangjuxu acupoints of the lower limbs from top to bottom, and press and knead the Taichong acupoint on the back of the foot with the vertical-pressing and kneading method.

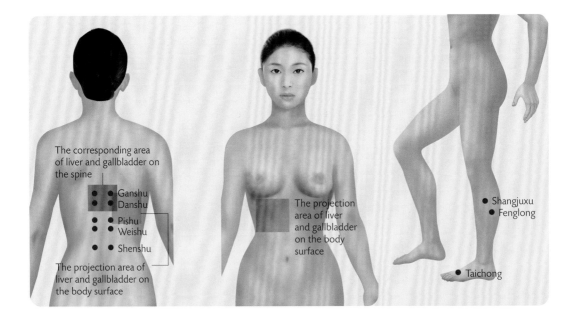

The corresponding area of liver and gallbladder on the spine

Ganshu
Danshu
Pishu
Weishu
Shenshu

The projection area of liver and gallbladder on the body surface

The projection area of liver and gallbladder on the body surface

Shangjuxu
Fenglong

Taichong

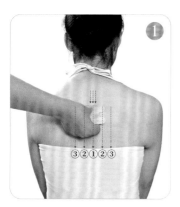
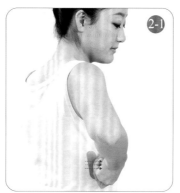
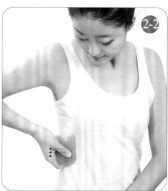

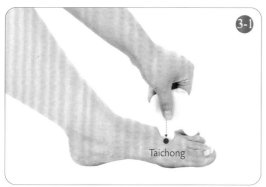
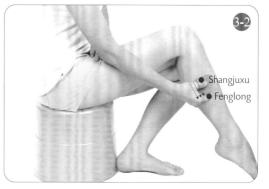

Expert Tip: Eye Bags Are a Sign of Spleen *Qi* Deficiency

Gua Sha treatment for eye bags begins with regulating the function of the spleen and stomach. The tonifying method is used to scrape loose and wrinkled under-eye bags. The scraping time for each area should be short. The liver, spleen, and kidney need to be regulated for full and swollen eye bags.

Bags under the eyes are the external manifestations of a deficiency of spleen *qi* and a deficiency of *qi* in the middle *jiao*. Tonifying the middle *jiao* and replenishing *qi*, and strengthening the spleen and stomach can prevent, slow down, and reduce bags under the eyes, and can also prolong life.

Human *qi* and blood come from the essence of food and drink created by the spleen and stomach. When *qi* and blood are sufficient, the complexion will be rosy, the muscles will be full and firm, and the skin and hair will be shiny and moist. Pathogens will not enter easily, and the body will not be prone to disease. Conversely, if the spleen and stomach are working abnormally and the transformation source of *qi* and blood is insufficient, the complexion will appear pale and sallow, and the muscles will be thin and slack. The hair will be shriveled and dull, and will thin and break easily. The body becomes susceptible to external pathogens, and there's a tendency to develop diseases easily, resulting in a shrinking body shape. As long as the normal transportation and transformation functions of the spleen and stomach can be maintained, aging can be delayed.

Diet Therapy and Skin Care for Reducing Eye Bags

Spleen-invigorating food includes japonica rice, glutinous rice, sago, sweet potato, coix seed, cowpea, white kidney beans, Chinese dates, Gorgon fruit, lotus seeds, peanuts, chestnuts, lotus root, and shiitake mushrooms.

To remove eye bags, you should increase your intake of high-quality protein (more than 90 grams every day), and eat more lean meat, milk, eggs, and aquatic products that are rich in high-quality protein.

You should also increase your intake of vitamins A and E. Vitamin A can promote vision, while vitamin E has a nourishing effect on the skin around the eyes. Foods rich in vitamin A include animal liver, butter, eggs, alfalfa, carrots, and apricots. Food rich in vitamin E includes sesame, peanuts, walnuts, and sunflower seeds.

At the same time, you should consume plenty of iron-rich food, because iron is the core component of hemoglobin. Iron-rich food includes animal liver, kelp, and lean meat. You should also eat food rich in vitamin C, such as wild jujubes, prickly pears, oranges, tomatoes, and green vegetables, because vitamin C can promote iron absorption.

Also, avoid drinking and smoking. Smoking will put the skin cells in a state of hypoxia, which will lead to the formation of bags under the eyes. Drinking alcohol will temporarily dilate the blood vessels and make the face flushed. It also makes the blood vessels shrink very quickly, especially near the bags under the eyes, temporarily causing ischemia and hypoxia around the eyes. If you drink alcohol over a long period of time, obvious bags will form under your eyes.

Food Therapy Recipe

Beef and cabbage soup: Take 500 grams of cabbage, 60 grams of beef, a little ginger and a little salt. Wash and cut the beef into thin slices, and put them into a pot with the ginger; add an appropriate amount of water and boil. Then put in the washed and cut cabbage and cook until the vegetables are cooked and the meat is tender. This recipe can invigorate the spleen and stomach, replenish *qi*, and dredge collaterals. Beef is warm in nature and rich in protein, and can remove excess water vapor from the body. Coupled with cabbage's ability to dredge the meridians, the blood will no longer stagnate in the local area, and the eye bags will naturally be eliminated.

Eye Masks

The best time to apply an eye mask is one week after your menstrual period, when the estrogen secretion in the body is strong, the metabolism speeds up, and the absorption capacity improves. At this time, applying an eye mask is the most effective; while taking a bath, applying it simultaneously can further accelerate circulation. After exercising, your metabolism will increase, which can accelerate the absorption of nutrients from the eye mask. Apply the eye mask before bed. Have a good night's sleep, and the nutrients will work as you rest, making the mask more effective.

How to apply eye cream: The skin around the eyes is very delicate. If eye cream is not used properly, it will not just fail to reduce fine lines, but may deepen them. First use the ring finger of your right hand to take some cream the size of half a grain of rice. Dot it under your right eye, and gently pull down the lower eyelid of the right eye with your left hand. This will smooth out the fine lines around the eyes and allow the eye cream to penetrate into these fine lines. Use the ring finger of your right hand to slowly massage the entire eye area clockwise 4 to 5 times from the lower right corner of the right eye until fully absorbed. Repeat on the left eye. Finally, use the ring fingers of both hands to gently pat the corresponding eyes, especially the bags, to help blood circulation and reduce the formation of dark circles and bags.

You can also make your own all-natural eye masks:

• Tea eye mask: Soak some tea leaves (green tea is the best) in hot water; let it cool down, soak it onto cotton pads, and apply to the eyes for 15 minutes, twice a week.

• Milk eye mask: Soak cotton pads in chilled skimmed milk and place them on the eyelids twice a day, for 10 minutes each time.

CHAPTER NINE
Eliminating Blue Veins and Redness

Under normal circumstances, blue veins and redness should not be seen on the facial skin. This is because they indicate a problem with the blood vessels in the face, caused by poor circulation due to insufficient blood flow or increased resistance to blood flow in the local or distal blood vessels. If there is a venous blood return obstacle in the capillaries, the blood color will be relatively dark, and blue blood vessels will be seen on the surface of the skin. More obvious blue veins on the head and face are usually a sign of increased pressure on the blood vessels in the head and poor blood circulation. Redness are caused by the persistent expansion of capillaries in the skin. It is characterized by the formation of red or purplish-red patches, dots, and lines of damage to the capillary network on the cheeks, with occasional burning or tingling sensations, and is more common in women.

Note: Some acupoints involved in this book are distributed symmetrically on both sides of the body. When conducting facial *gua sha*, except for a few acupoints that require one-sided scraping, the rest are all symmetrical acupoints on both sides of the body by default.

Key Points of the Technique

1. Apply facial *gua sha* cream on the treatment area first.

2. Redness mostly appear on the cheeks and cheekbones, and cannot be scraped directly. Use the pushing and scraping method to carefully find and eliminate the positive reaction areas at the Quanliao acupoints.

3. Blue veins are a manifestation of internal blood vessel stasis, so the source and cause must be found. You should look for pain sensitive points on the upper, lower, left, and right sides of the veins, and scrape there. The thicker the veins are, the deeper the stasis is. The pressure should penetrate under the skin and between the soft tissue in the muscles. Look for pain sensitive points and other positive reactions.

Blue Veins on the Forehead

Protruding blue veins in the middle of the forehead indicate long-term fatigue, tension, and poor blood circulation in the head and neck. Protruding blue veins on both sides of the forehead and temples indicate *qi* and blood stasis in the liver and gallbladder, and poor blood circulation, mostly related to excessive

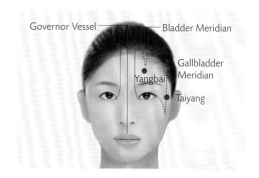

mental stress, and may cause dizziness and headache. When blue veins protrude and twist, this can be a sign of high blood pressure and cerebral arteriosclerosis.

Facial Beauty *Gua Sha*

1. Clean the face and apply facial *gua sha* cream. Scrape the Governor Vessel, the Bladder Meridian in the middle of the forehead, the Gallbladder Meridian on both sides, the Yangbai acupoint, and the Taiyang acupoint area with the pushing and scraping method. Focus on scraping the areas above, below, to the left, and to the right of the blue veins. Scrape each area 5 times, looking for positive reactions such as gravel, nodules, and pain.

   2. Use the pushing and scraping method and the kneading and scraping method to focus on the forehead meridians, acupoints, Yangbai acupoints, Taiyang acupoints, and the positive reaction areas under the vicinity of the blue veins 10 times.

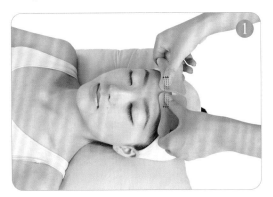 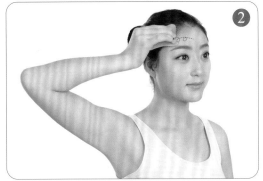

Consolidating *Gua Sha* on the Head, Hands, and Feet

1. Use the sharp-edge scraping method to scrape the mid-frontal belt and the first lateral-frontal belt and the second lateral-frontal belt on both sides of the head.

   2. Use a scraping comb to scrape the top of the head, the Governor Vessel and the Bladder Meridian on the back of the head, and the Gallbladder Meridian on the side of the head with the surface-scraping method.

   3. Use a scraper to scrape the brain area on the middle finger and the head area on the feet with the surface-scraping method until the skin feels warm.

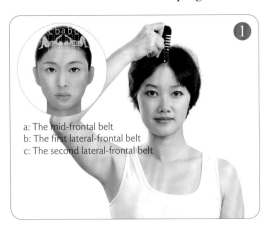

a: The mid-frontal belt
b: The first lateral-frontal belt
c: The second lateral-frontal belt

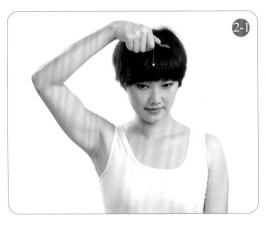

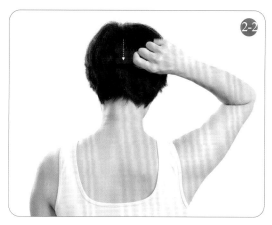

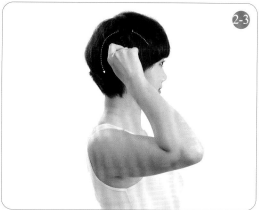

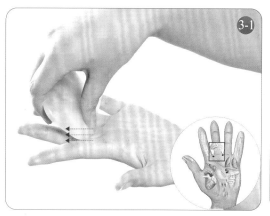

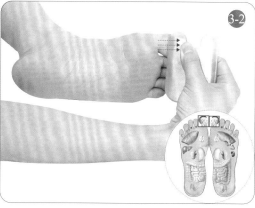

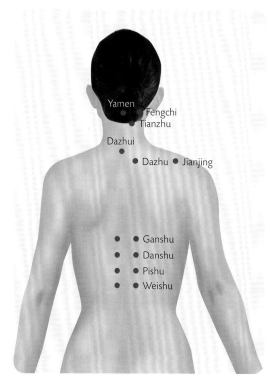

Yamen
Fengchi
Tianzhu
Dazhui
Dazhu • Jianjing
Ganshu
Danshu
Pishu
Weishu

Whole-Body *Gua Sha* and Conditioning

1. Apply scraping oil on the cervical spine. ① First, scrape the Governor Vessel in the middle of the cervical spine, and use surface-scraping from the Yamen acupoint to the Dazhui acupoint. ② Then, scrape the Bladder Meridian via the Tianzhu acupoint to the Dazhu acupoint. ③ Finally, scrape from the Gallbladder Meridian through the Fengchi acupoint to the Jianjing acupoint.

2. Use the surface-scraping method to scrape the Ganshu, Danshu, Pishu, and Weishu acupoints on the back from top to bottom.

3. Press and knead the Taichong acupoint on the foot with the vertical-pressing and kneading method.

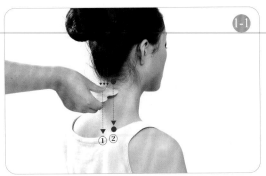

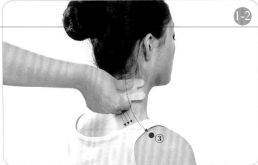

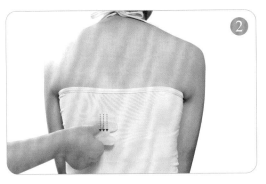

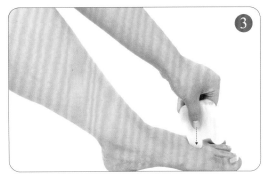

Expert Tip: Why Blue Veins Occur

When the superficial veins dilate, blue veins will appear on the skin. When a person is angry or excited, their heartbeat speeds up, quickly causing major congestion in the arteries and veins. Expansion of the subcutaneous veins can be seen, causing visible blue veins to bulge. This is normal. As people grow older, blood flow slows down and the elasticity of the blood vessels decreases. The skin becomes thinner, and subcutaneous fat decreases. Blue veins will appear on the back of the hands, upper limbs, and lower limbs. The elasticity of blood vessels decreases with age, if there are diseases such as high cholesterol, high blood sugar, high blood pressure, or liver and kidney diseases, the blood circulation will be hindered, and the venous blood return will be blocked. When the pressure increases, the blue veins in some parts will gradually increase. They will become more and more obvious, even raised, varicose, distorted, and deepened in color.

In TCM, it is thought that the protruding veins are actually caused by poor flow of *qi* and blood in the meridians. Veins that are obviously protruding and becoming thicker and twisted, are caused by stagnation in the body. If there is stool in the gastrointestinal tract, the long-term accumulation of toxins will harm the body, or cause phlegm, dampness, blood stasis, and stagnation of *qi* in the meridians, and blue veins will appear on certain parts of the body surface. Obvious blue veins are an external reflection of waste in the body. The more veins there are in each area, and the more obviously they are raised and twisted, the more stagnation there is in the body.

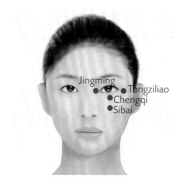

Blue Veins around the Eyes

In women, visible blue veins in the inner corner of the eye and lower eyelid are symptoms of insufficient kidney *qi*, irregular menstruation, gynecological problems, and spleen and stomach deficiency-cold. Blue veins located under the outer corners of the eyes indicate that there is a stagnation of *qi* and blood in the meridians in the shoulders.

Facial Beauty *Gua Sha*

1. After cleansing the skin, apply facial *gua sha* cream. Press and knead the Jingming acupoint with the vertical-pressing and kneading method; scrape the Chengqi, Sibai, and Tongziliao acupoints with the pushing and scraping method, and focus on the lower eyelid and positive reactions in the form of gritty nodules. Scrape each area 5 times.

2. Press and knead the lower eyelid and the positive reaction points near the blue veins with the flat-pressing and kneading method. Scrape each area 5 times.

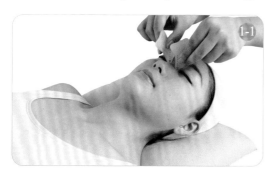
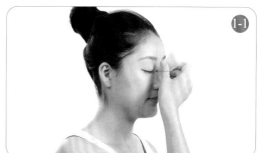
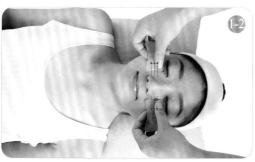
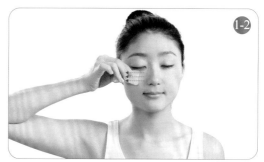
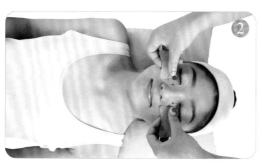
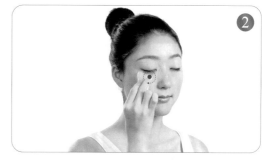

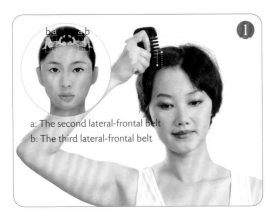

a: The second lateral-frontal belt
b: The third lateral-frontal belt

Consolidating *Gua Sha* on the Head, Hands, and Feet

1. Use the sharp-edge scraping method to scrape the second lateral-frontal belt and the third lateral-frontal belt on both sides of the head.

2. Use the scraper to scrape the thenar and hypothenar on the hands, gonad area in the sole and on the inner and outer sides of the heels.

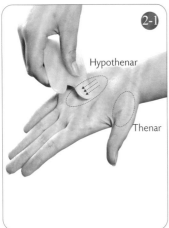

Hypothenar

Thenar

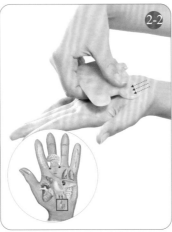

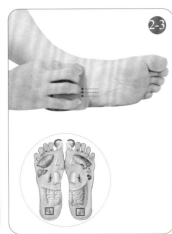

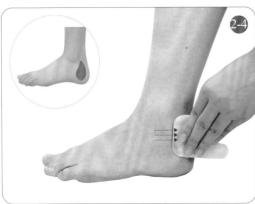

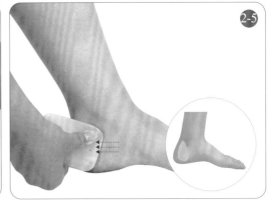

Whole-Body *Gua Sha* and Conditioning

1. Use the surface-scraping method to scrape the Mingmen, Geshu, Pishu, Weishu, Shenshu, Zhishi, and Baliao acupoints on the back and waist from top to bottom.

2. Use the surface-scraping method to scrape the projection area of uterus and ovary on the lower abdomen from top to bottom, focusing on the Qihai acupoint to the Guanyuan acupoint.

3. Use the surface-scraping method to scrape the Xuehai and Sanyinjiao acupoints on the lower limbs from top to bottom.

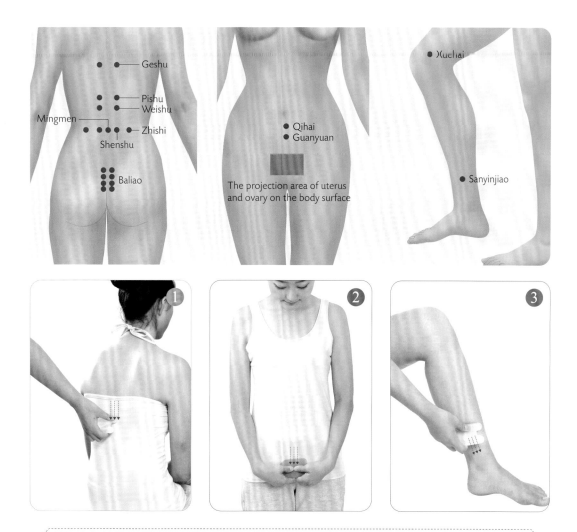

The projection area of uterus and ovary on the body surface

Expert Tip: Love Life and Age Slower

Facial appearance is an outward display of the health of the viscera and organs. As we grow older, our appearance will change. As well as recording changes in the viscera, our faces also mirror the fluctuations in our mental journey. No matter how old they are, a person who loves life and is full of positive and optimistic emotions will have a facial appearance that displays a sense of harmonious and tranquil beauty.

We are often confused by our complex and diverse lifestyles, controlled and attracted invisibly by so many external things, and placed under great pressure. We therefore forget to enjoy the present. In my daily clinical work, I often meet highly successful women who put too much of a burden on themselves in their careers, damaging their appearance and even their health. While performing *gua sha* and conditioning for them, I encourage them not only to love their career and family, but also to love themselves and look after their bodies and minds. True, natural beauty cannot be conferred by any external method.

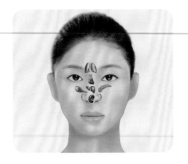

Blue Veins on the Nose

Blue veins at the root of the nose indicate gastrointestinal accumulation. Children with blue veins here are prone to colds, gastrointestinal diseases, and indigestion. Blue veins on the bridge of the nose indicate incoordination between the liver and spleen, gastrointestinal stagnation, stomach pain, abdominal distension, and indigestion.

Facial Beauty *Gua Sha*

1. Clean the face and apply facial *gua sha* cream. Scrape the lung area and the heart area between the eyebrows, the root of the nose to the tip of the nose with the pushing and scraping method; focus on the liver and gallbladder areas, and the upper, lower, left, and right areas of blue veins. Scrape each area 5 times, looking for positive reactions such as gravel, nodules, and pain.

2. Use the pushing and scraping method and flat-kneading and scraping method to scrape the nose and the positive reaction areas under the vicinity of the blue veins 10 times.

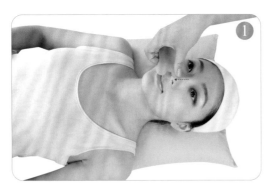
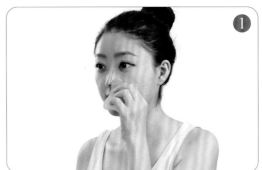
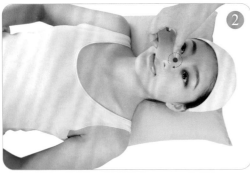
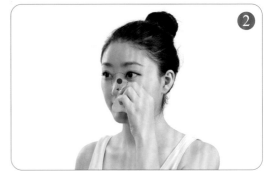

Consolidating *Gua Sha* on the Head, Hands, and Feet

1. Use the sharp-edge scraping method to scrape the mid-frontal belt and the front and middle one-third area of the frontal belt of the head top.

2. Use the scraper to scrape the thenar and hypothenar of the hands, and the liver, stomach, and intestine areas in the sole with the pushing and scraping method.

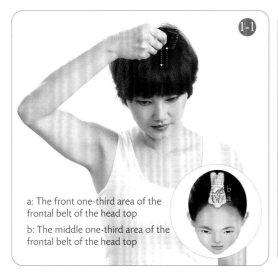

1-1

a: The front one-third area of the frontal belt of the head top
b: The middle one-third area of the frontal belt of the head top

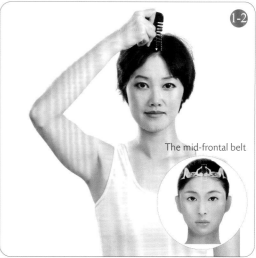

1-2

The mid-frontal belt

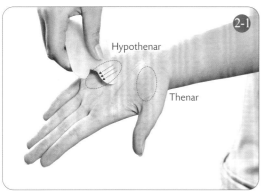

2-1

Hypothenar

Thenar

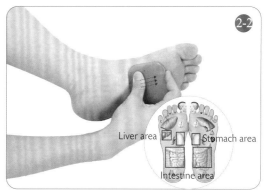

2-2

Liver area   Stomach area

Intestine area

Whole-Body *Gua Sha* and Conditioning

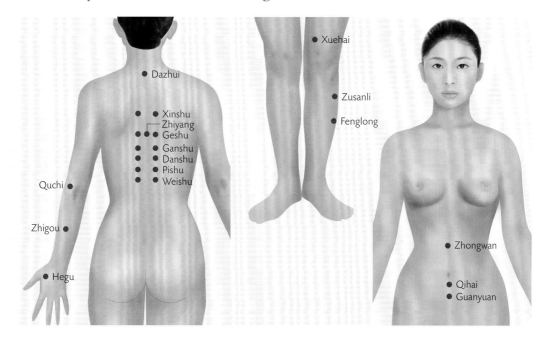

Xuehai

Dazhui

Zusanli

Xinshu
Zhiyang
Geshu
Ganshu
Danshu
Pishu
Weishu

Fenglong

Quchi

Zhigou

Zhongwan

Qihai
Guanyuan

Hegu

1. Use the surface-scraping method to scrape the Dazhui acupoint to the Zhiyang, Xinshu, Geshu, Ganshu, Danshu, Pishu, and Weishu acupoints on the back and waist.

2. Use the surface-scraping method to scrape the Zhongwan, Qihai, and Guanyuan acupoints on the abdomen from top to bottom.

3. Use the surface-scraping method to scrape the Quchi acupoint in the upper limbs from top to bottom; press and knead the Hegu and Zhigou acupoints with the flat-pressing and kneading method; use the surface-scraping method to scrape the Zusanli acupoint to the Fenglong and Xuehai acupoints in the lower limbs from top to bottom.

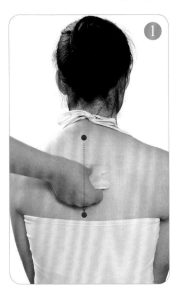
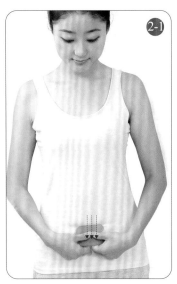
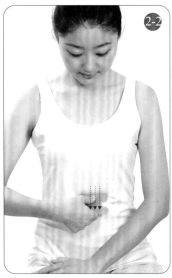
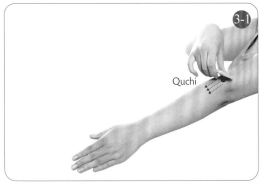
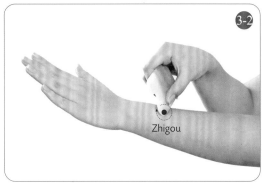
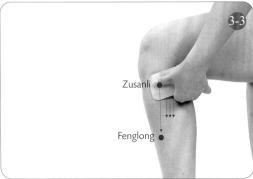
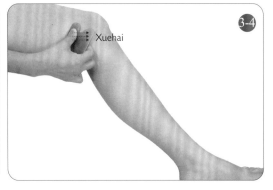

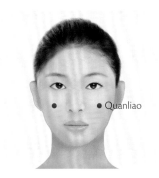

Quanliao

Quanliao

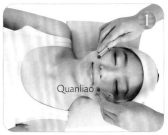

Quanliao

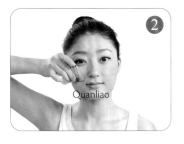

Quanliao

Redness in the Center of the Cheek Areas

The appearance of redness on the cheekbones may be related to genetics or environmental factors. It is common in plateau climates. Due to the lack of oxygen in the mountains, the amount of hemoglobin in the blood increases. In addition to strong ultraviolet radiation, the dry climate can damage the stratum corneum, resulting in poor capillary dilation or even rupture of the capillaries, causing redness. In addition to genetic and environmental factors, mild redness usually indicate heart-*qi* deficiency and heart-blood stasis.

Facial Beauty *Gua Sha*

1. Clean the face, then find the exact location of the Quanliao acupoint, which is directly below the outer canthus of the eye, at the depression of the lower edge of the zygomatic bone. Apply facial *gua sha* cream, then scrape the Quanliao acupoint from the bottom upward with the pushing and scraping method, avoiding the blood streaks. Look for painful, gravelly positive reaction points, and scrape 5 to 10 times according to the severity of the pain.

   2. Use the pushing and scraping method or the

flat-pressing and kneading method, avoiding redness. Scrape the positive reaction points under the Quanliao acupoint 5 times.

Consolidating *Gua Sha* on the Head, Hands, and Feet

1. Use the sharp-edge scraping method to scrape the first lateral-frontal belt and the second lateral-frontal belt on both sides of the head.

2. Scrape the thenar and hypothenar of the hand, the heart area and the intestine area in the sole, with the pushing and scraping method.

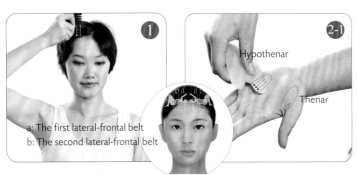
a: The first lateral-frontal belt
b: The second lateral-frontal belt

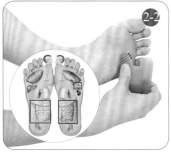

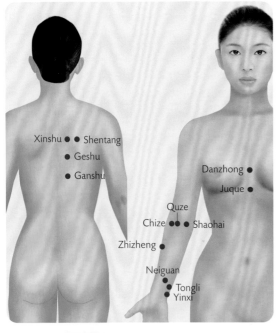

Whole-Body *Gua Sha* and Conditioning

1. Use the surface-scraping method to scrape Xinshu, Shentang, Geshu, and Ganshu acupoints on both sides of the back.

2. Use the single-angle scraping method to scrape from the Danzhong acupoint to the Juque acupoint from top to bottom.

3. Use the surface-scraping method to scrape the Yinxi, Tongli, Neiguan, and Zhizheng acupoints from top to bottom. Use the clapping method to pat the Chize, Quze, and Shaohai acupoints in the fossa of the elbow.

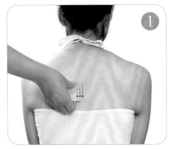

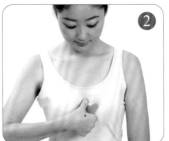

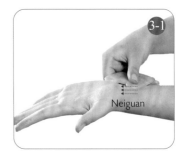

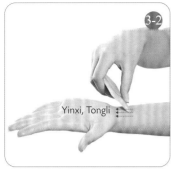

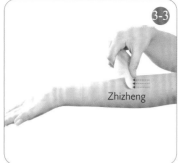

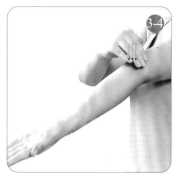

Yinxi, Tongli

Zhizheng

Expert Tip: Treatment and Care of Red Blood Streaks

Red blood streaks or redness on the face are caused by the dilation of capillaries or the fact that some capillaries are located close to the surface. People with redness have thinner facial skin, which is redder than normal skin. Some only have redness on both sides of the cheeks, with a round border.

Redness are related to the blood circulation system, which can be affected by wind, sun exposure, high temperatures, dry air damage, and the facial meridians, resulting in dilation of the capillaries, causing illnesses. Blood stasis within can also block the meridians leading to poor blood circulation. The stagnated blood can also block the skin, expanding the blood vessels. Poor blood circulation makes it difficult for toxins to be excreted from the body, leading to the formation of redness.

No matter the cause of the redness, they are always related to poor blood circulation at the Quanliao acupoint and the stagnation of *qi* and blood in the meridians. The Quanliao acupoint is the point of the Small Intestine Meridian. In TCM it is believed that the heart and small intestine are related. Deficiency of the heart *qi* directly affects the *qi* operation of the Small Intestine Meridian. When the Small Intestine Meridian has insufficient energy, there will be a stagnation of *qi* and blood at the important node of the Quanliao acupoint, and redness will appear on the skin. Therefore, people with redness will experience obvious pain or positive reactions such as gravel and nodules at this point. After repeated scraping, the stasis points are slowly dredged, redness can be relieved, and slight redness will disappear. However, it must be combined with tonifying heart *qi*, and promoting blood circulation to remove blood stasis on relevant parts of the body at the same time, in order to consolidate the effect of facial *gua sha*.

Skin care for redness is also very important. Drink plenty of water and moisturize the skin. Use moisturizing skin care products without alcohol, fragrance, and preservatives, and do not exfoliate too regularly. UV rays from the sun will make redness worse, so cover them properly to reduce external stimulation. Wash your face with warm water as much as possible. Do not alternate with cold and hot water, as this can cause the pores to expand and shrink quickly, dilating the capillaries and aggravating facial redness.

Protrusion of Sublingual Veins

When you roll up the tip of your tongue, you will see two thick veins underneath it. The sublingual veins correspond to the coronary arteries of the human body. If these two veins are dark purple or black, bulging, or twisted like a snake, it indicates poor blood circulation in the heart, and possibly coronary heart disease. Cardiovascular and cerebrovascular diseases, hemorrhoids, and some gynecological diseases will also cause danger signals to appear in the sublingual veins.

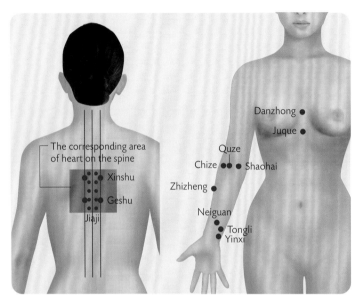

Facial Beauty *Gua Sha*

1. Use the surface-scraping method to scrape the corresponding area of heart on the spine. ① First, use the surface-scraping method to scrape the Governor Vessel between the 4th and 8th thoracic vertebrae on the back. ② Use the dual-angle method to scrape the Jiaji acupoints from top to bottom on both sides of the same horizontal section of the Governor Vessel. ③ Then, use the surface-scraping method to scrape the 3-cun wide area on both sides of the Governor Vessel from top to bottom. Focus on scraping the Xinshu and Geshu acupoints on both sides of the back.

2. Use the single angle-scraping method to scrape from the Danzhong acupoint to the Juque acupoint from top to bottom.

3. Use the surface-scraping method to scrape the Yinxi, Tongli, Neiguan, and Zhizheng acupoints from top to bottom. Use the clapping method to pat the Chize, Quze, and Shaohai acupoints in the fossa of the elbow.

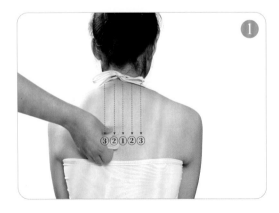

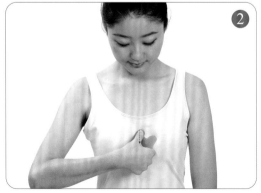

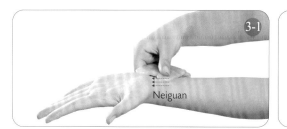
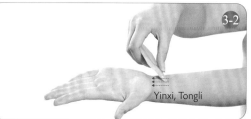
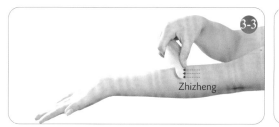
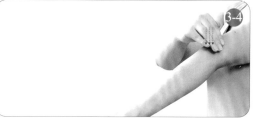

Expert Tip: Check Your Sublingual Vein for Cardiovascular Health

Observing changes in the sublingual veins is an important part of TCM tongue diagnosis. Since these veins are visible and not covered by skin, it is easy to obtain relevant information about blood oxygen saturation, blood viscosity, and blood volume about the body, which is very useful in assessing its health condition. With cardiovascular and cerebrovascular diseases, the sublingual veins will appear dark purple, distended, or twisted. People who are over 45 years old should look out for the following conditions:

Dark purple sublingual veins: This can be a sign of arteriosclerosis. As the degree of purpleness and darkness increases, the severity of arteriosclerosis increases accordingly. There may also be fundus arteriosclerosis, headache, dizziness, and memory loss.

Distended sublingual veins: If the sublingual veins are dark purple and also distended and flexed, this can be a sign of high blood pressure and arteriosclerosis. If the flexion is severe, protruding out of the tongue like an earthworm, and the condition is serious, often accompanied by a headache, dizziness, and irritability, attention should be paid to changes in blood pressure. If the veins under the tongue are purple and dark, with nodules as small as a grain of rice, or as big as a grain of corn, be wary of arteriosclerosis and coronary heart disease.

Protruding and distended sublingual veins must not be underestimated. You should undergo relevant tests immediately and have regular medical check-ups. People with severe sublingual vein problems should use *gua sha* therapy as well as take medication for comprehensive regulation. Patients with severe heart disease should be careful when having *gua sha* therapy on the chest and back. The strergth exerted should gradually increase from light to heavy, and clapping should not be used on the elbow fossa meridian and acupoints to avoid pain stimulation-induced heart disease.

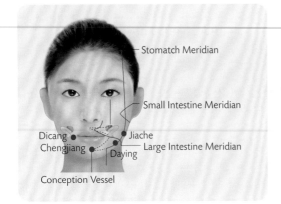

- Stomatch Meridian
- Small Intestine Meridian
Dicang
Chengjiang
Jiache
Daying
Large Intestine Meridian
Conception Vessel

Blue Veins on the Lower Jaw

Blue veins on the lower jaw are a sign of rheumatism in the lower limbs, lower *jiao* deficiency-cold, or blood stasis, often accompanied by excessive leukorrhea, fatigue, weak waist and knees, knee joint pain, or cold hands and feet.

Facial Beauty *Gua Sha*

1. Clean the face and apply facial *gua sha* cream. Scrape the Chengjiang acupoint on the lower jaw with the pushing and scraping method. Scrape the Dicang and Daying acupoints at the corner of the mouth, the facial lower limb area, and the Jiache acupoint from the inside to the outside and upwards, focusing on the upper, lower, left, and right sides of the blue veins. Scrape each part 5 times, looking for positive reactions such as gravel, nodules, and pain. Use the pushing and scraping method or kneading and scraping method to focus on the positive reaction areas under the lower jaw, lower limb area, and the parts near the blue veins 10 times.

2. Use the groove of the scraper to scrape the Conception Vessel under the jaw with the pushing and scraping method, and scrape the Stomach Meridian, Large Intestine Meridian, and Small Intestine Meridian on both sides, and scrape each part 10 times. Use the surface-scraping method to scrape down the middle and two sides of the front neck.

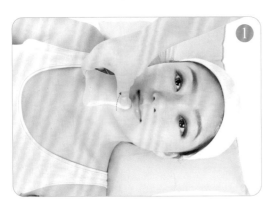

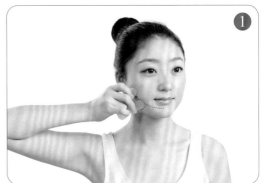

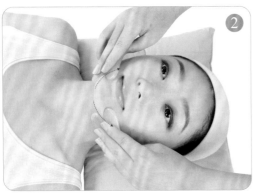

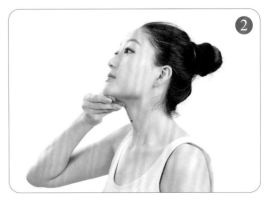

Consolidating *Gua Sha* on the Head, Hands, and Feet

1. Use the sharp edge scraping method to scrape the middle and rear one-third areas of the frontal belt of the head top, and the upper one-third area of the anterior and posterior oblique belt of the parieto-temporal region.

    2. Scrape the kidney area and the uterus area on the hand, and the gonad area inside and outside the heel and in the sole, with the pushing and scraping method.

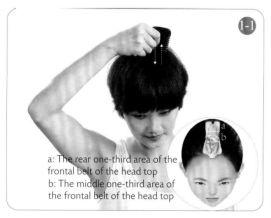

a: The rear one-third area of the frontal belt of the head top
b: The middle one-third area of the frontal belt of the head top

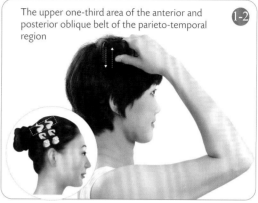

The upper one-third area of the anterior and posterior oblique belt of the parieto-temporal region

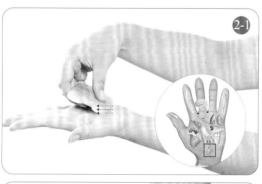

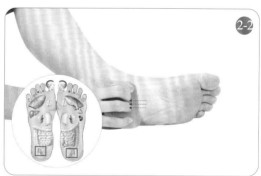

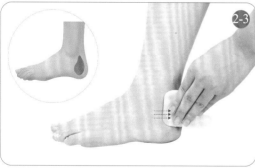

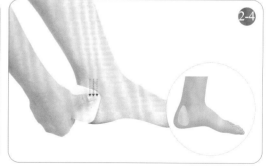

Whole-Body *Gua Sha* and Conditioning

1. Use the surface-scraping method to scrape the Mingmen, Shenshu, Zhishi, and Baliao acupoints on the back from top to bottom.

    2. Use the surface-scraping method to scrape the projection area of uterus and ovary on the lower abdomen from top to bottom, focusing on the Qihai acupoint to the Guanyuan acupoint.

3. Use the clapping method to tap the Weizhong, Weiyang, and Yin'gu acupoints on the lower limbs. Use the surface-scraping method to scrape the Xiyangguan, Yanglingquan, and Zusanli acupoints on the lower limbs from top to bottom.

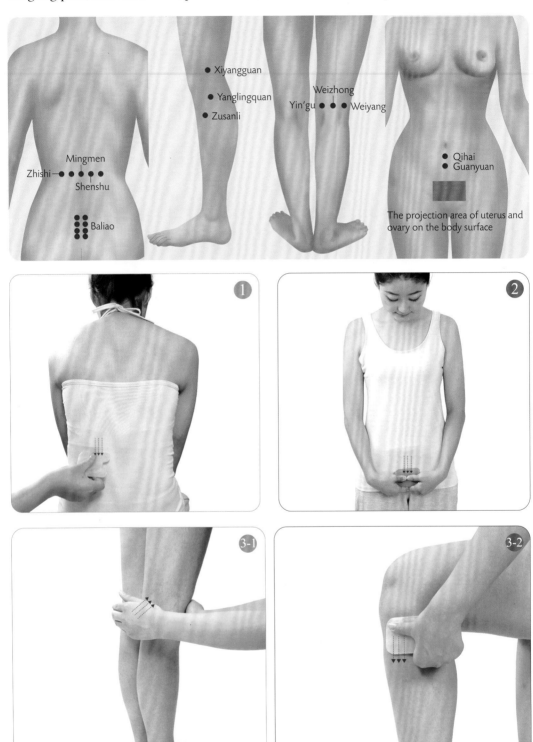

Xiyangguan

Yanglingquan

Zusanli

Weizhong

Yin'gu ● ● ● Weiyang

Mingmen

Zhishi ● ● ● ● Shenshu

Baliao

Qihai
Guanyuan

The projection area of uterus and ovary on the body surface

❶

❷

❸-1

❸-2

Diet Therapy and Skin Care

In terms of diet, be careful not to eat too much spicy food or food that is irritating to the skin, and do not drink alcohol. Alcohol has a drying effect, which is particularly bad for sensitive skin. Eat food that is rich in B vitamins, such as oatmeal.

Food Therapy Recipes

• Chrysanthemum tea: The chrysanthemum used should be chamomile, as it isn't bitter. Make tea with about 3 grams each time, drink 3 times a day. You can also boil chrysanthemum, honeysuckle, and licorice together and consume as a substitute for tea. It can calm the liver and improve eyesight, clearing away heat and detoxifying. They can also lower blood pressure, relieve stress, help reduce blood vessel pressure, and reduce redness.

    • Chrysanthemum porridge: Take 15 grams of chrysanthemum, and 100 grams of japonica rice. First grind the chrysanthemum into a fine powder and set aside. Clean the japonica rice and put it into a pot. Add an appropriate amount of water, bring to a boil over high heat, then turn to a low heat and cook until it is half-done, then add finely chopped chrysanthemums. Continue to cook over a low heat until the rice has softened into porridge. Eat twice a day, in the morning and evening, to reduce redness.

    • Kelp and mung bean soup: Take 150 grams of kelp, soaked, washed, and chopped; 150 grams of mung beans, washed. Boil in a pot until thoroughly cooked, then mix with brown sugar. Drink twice a day. Mung beans clear away heat and detoxify, and kelp reduces blood vessel pressure. Cooking them together can significantly improve facial redness and red blood streaks.

    • Fresh celery juice: Wash 200 grams of celery, scald it in boiling water for 2 minutes, chop it, then squeeze it through gauze. Add sugar to taste, and drink twice a day. Celery can lower blood pressure, calm the liver, induce calmness, relieve spasms, stop vomiting, and promote diuresis. It significantly improves dizziness, headaches, facial flushing, and protruding blue veins.

Homemade Face Masks

• Aloe and egg white mask: Take 1 piece of aloe vera leaf, egg white, and a little honey. Mix the aloe vera pulp with the egg white and honey. Apply it on red blood streaks for 10 minutes, and then wash it off with warm water. Aloe vera has moisturizing, anti-inflammatory, freckle-removing, sun-protective, and wound-healing effects. Using this mask can inhibit the formation of redness.

    • Rose and vitamin E mask: Put rose petals into a pot and add distilled water or mineral water. Cook for 1 hour on a high heat, and then strain the juice; break a vitamin E capsule to extract the oil, and add it to the rose juice; apply it to the redness with a small cotton swab. Vitamin E can fully moisturize dry and red skin in autumn and winter, and rose has astringent, calming, and fading effects on redness.

CHAPTER TEN
Beautifying and Moisturizing the Lips

The health of the spleen and stomach can be reflected in the lips. If the spleen's function of transforming *qi* and blood is normal, the lips should be bright, moist, and pale red. Brightness means sufficient spleen and stomach *qi*, and moistness means sufficient essence, blood, and body fluids. There are four meridians around the mouth. The Large Intestine Meridian wraps around the upper lip and intersects in the middle. The left branch goes to the right, and the right branch goes to the left, distributed on both sides of the nostrils, connecting with the Stomach Meridian, so the skin of the upper lip and the area around it belong to the large intestine. The Stomach Meridian starts from the Yingxiang acupoint on each side of the nose, enters the upper gum and exits through the Dicang acupoint. It surrounds the lips, and meets Chengjiang acupoint downwards in the chin-labial groove, then goes to the Daying acupoint. The lower lip and the skin around it belong to the stomach. If the upper lip is too thin, it indicates that the function of the large intestine is weak. A balance between the upper and lower lips is better. The middle of each lip is also connected to the Governor Vessel and the Conception Vessel respectively, reflecting the fluctuations of *yin* and *yang* in the body.

Healthy lips should be light red, shiny, round and full, with no dryness, ulcers, cracks, or coldsores. The color of the lips will vary due to factors such as age, constitution, genetics, nutrition, living habits, or *qi* and blood diseases of the viscera. Lips not only reveal the health of the viscera, but also the aging process. Lip color, including the color of the skin around the lips, reflects the current *qi* and blood health of the viscera.

Note: Some acupoints involved in this book are distributed symmetrically on both sides of the body. When conducting facial *gua sha*, except for a few acupoints that require one-sided scraping, the rest are all symmetrical acupoints on both sides of the body by default.

Key Points of the Technique

1. The lip beautification and moisturizing scraping method involves scraping the skin of the upper and lower lips and the exposed red mucous membrane tissue. When scraping the skin of the upper and lower lips, the flat surface of the tool should touch the skin at an angle of 0 degrees. When scraping the exposed red mucous membrane, the tool should be completely in contact with the membrane, and the scraping area should not exceed the range of daily lipstick application. The lines where the skin meets the red mucous membrane are the key parts for scraping.

2. Apply facial *gua sha* cream on the treatment area first, and wipe off with a wet tissue or wash off immediately after scraping.

3. Use the pushing and scraping method and flat-pressing and kneading method. The pressure should penetrate the soft tissue under the skin of the lips and among the muscles.

4. Scrape slowly, and controlled to scrape 2 to 3 times within one calm breath.

5. Scrape from the middle to the corners of the mouth on both sides in accordance with the direction of the lip muscles. When scraping the upper lip to the corners of the mouth, the pressure should be reduced appropriately. When scraping the lower lip to the corners of the mouth, the pressure should be increased appropriately to lift outward and upward.

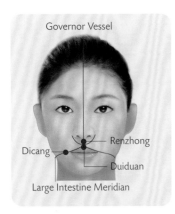

Governor Vessel

Renzhong

Dicang

Duiduan

Large Intestine Meridian

Pale, Bluish Upper Lip

A pale, bluish upper lip is a sign of deficiency-cold in the spleen, large intestine, and lower *jiao*. Those suffering from this will often display symptoms of fearing cold and preferring warmth, bloating, abdominal pain, constipation, or diarrhea. Women may suffer from menstrual pain, delayed menstruation, and purple menstrual blood, low flow, as well as leukorrhea that is thin and clear and in large quantity. Pale lips can also be a sign of anemia.

Facial Beauty *Gua Sha*

1. Clean the facial skin and lips. After applying facial *gua sha* cream, scrape the skin of the upper lip first. Use the pushing and scraping method to scrape the upper lip from the Renzhong acupoint to the Duiduan acupoint, and then push and scrape outwards from the Renzhong and Duiduan acupoints to the Dicang acupoint at the corner of the mouth. Push and scrape the Dicang acupoint from bottom to outer top, 5 times in total. Then use the flat-pressing and kneading method to scrape each point 5 times.

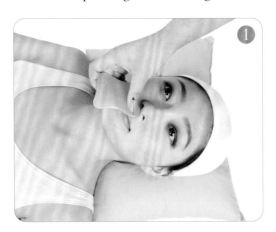

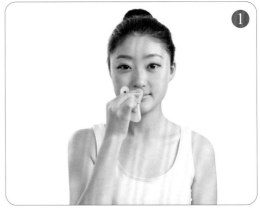

2. Scrape the red part of the upper lip. Place the scraper flat on the lip lines, and use the pushing and scraping method to scrape from the Duiduan acupoint at the tip of the middle of the upper lip to the outside along the upper lip lines to the corner of the mouth. Scrape 5 times. Scrape the Dicang acupoint 5 times with an upward and outward lifting force with the flat-pressing and kneading method.

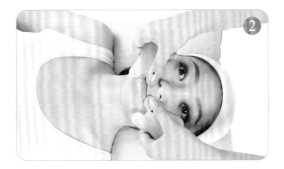
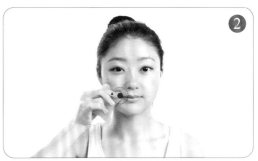

Consolidating *Gua Sha* on the Head, Hands, and Feet

1. Use the sharp-edge scraping method to scrape the second lateral-frontal belt and the third lateral-frontal belt on both sides of the head, and the middle and rear one-third area of the frontal belt of the head top.

2. Use the pushing and scraping method to scrape the thenar and hypothenar on the hands, and the gonad areas on the inner and outer sides of the heel and in the sole.

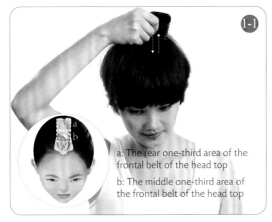

a: The rear one-third area of the frontal belt of the head top

b: The middle one-third area of the frontal belt of the head top

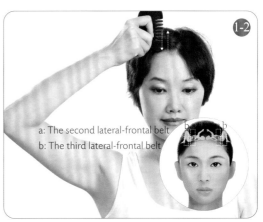

a: The second lateral-frontal belt
b: The third lateral-frontal belt

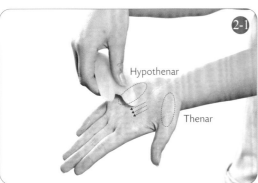

Hypothenar

Thenar

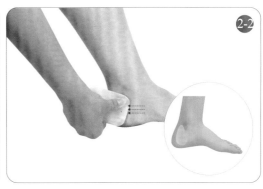

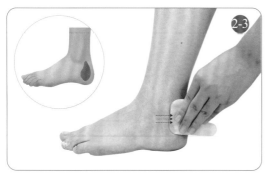

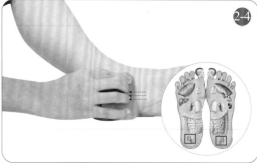

Whole-Body *Gua Sha* and Conditioning

1. Scrape the Mingmen, Shenshu, Zhishi, Dachangshu, Pangguangshu, and Baliao acupoints.

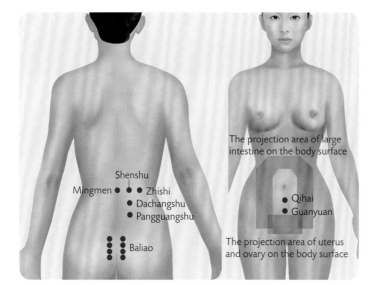

Shenshu
Mingmen ● ● ● Zhishi
● Dachangshu
● Pangguangshu

Baliao

The projection area of large intestine on the body surface

● Qihai
● Guanyuan

The projection area of uterus and ovary on the body surface

2. Use the surface-scraping method to scrape the projection areas of large intestine, uterus, and ovary on the abdomen from top to bottom, focusing on the Qihai acupoint to the Guanyuan acupoint.

3. Use the surface-scraping method to scrape the Zusanli, Gongsun, and Sanyinjiao acupoints of the lower limbs from top to bottom.

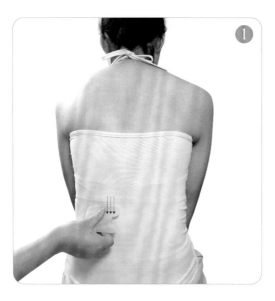

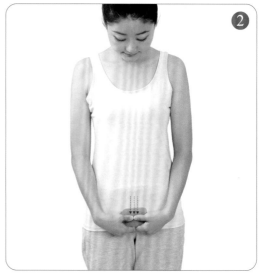

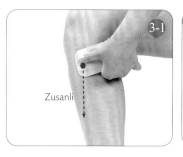

Zusanli

3-1

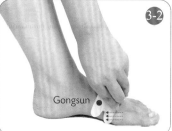

Gongsun

3-2

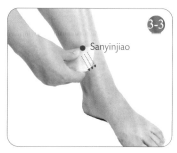

Sanyinjiao

3-3

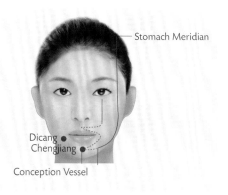

Stomach Meridian

Dicang
Chengjiang

Conception Vessel

Expert Tip: Observing Microcirculation through the Mouth and Lips

In the human body, blood flows through the distal ends of arteries, then into the capillaries, and then joins and flows into the beginning of the venules. The blood circulation in the capillaries between the arterioles and venules is called microcirculation. The basic function of microcirculation is to supply blood, energy, and nutrients to cells, and at the same time take away harmful metabolic waste such as lactic acid and carbon dioxide, so as to maintain good internal circulation and vitality. Microcirculation also plays the role of a "second heart," because it is impossible for the body to send blood from the heart to the tissue cells only by contraction force; it must be regulated by microvessels to perfuse the blood into the cells.

The quality of microcirculation is directly related to the quality of life. The lips are the best indicator of microcirculation, because they have no sweat glands, sebaceous glands, or hairs, meaning less interference and better transparency than the skin. The capillaries in the lips are quite abundant, and combined with the thin mucous membrane of the lips, they can clearly reflect the condition of the blood, including changes in *qi* and blood, oxygen content, and the quality of the blood. Slight changes to the body's internal environment can be detected timely by observing changes to the color of the lips.

Lip tissue are prone to dryness because they do not have sebaceous glands. Avoid licking your lips, as this can make the dryness worse. People with dry lips should drink plenty of water to increase their body fluids.

Pale Lower Lip

A pale lower lip is a symptom of stomach *qi* deficiency-cold, loss of appetite, and cold pain in the stomach, often accompanied by symptoms of *qi* deficiency, fatigue, lassitude, lack of appetite, and loose stools. Severe lower lip pallor is often associated with anemia or massive blood loss from various causes.

Facial Beauty *Gua Sha*

1. Clean the facial skin and lips. After applying facial *gua sha* cream, scrape the skin of the lower lip first. Use the pushing and scraping method to scrape from the Chengjiang acupoint on the lower jaw outward to the Dicang acupoint on the corner of the mouth, and scrape the Dicang acupoint from bottom to top outwards. Scrape 5 times each. Then use the flat-pressing and kneading method to scrape each point 5 times.

    2. Scrape the red part of the lower lip. Place the scraper flat on the lip lines, and use the pushing and scraping method to scrape from the middle of the lip outwards to the corner of the mouth, 5 times. Flat-press and knead the Dicang acupoint 5 times with an outward and upward lifting force.

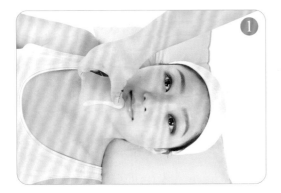

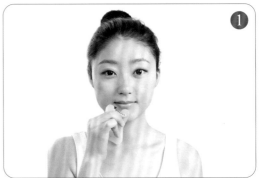

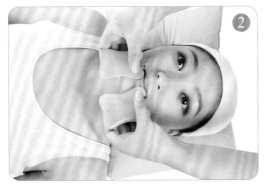

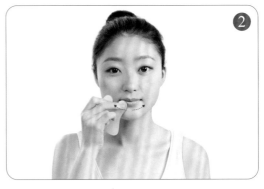

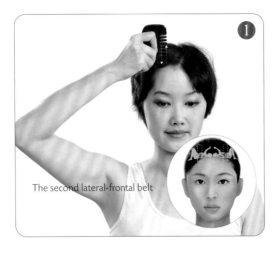

The second lateral-frontal belt

Consolidating *Gua Sha* on the Head, Hands, and Feet

1. Use the sharp-edge scraping method to scrape the second lateral-frontal belt on both sides of the head.

    2. Scrape the stomach area on the hands and feet with the pushing and scraping method.

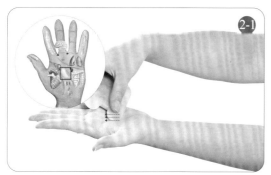

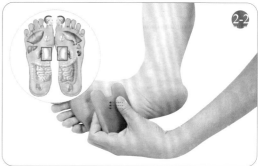

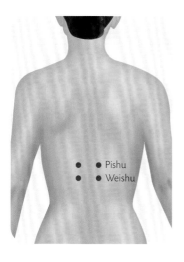

- Pishu
- Weishu

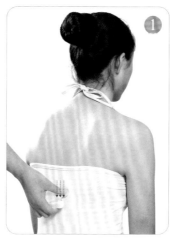

Whole-Body *Gua Sha* and Conditioning

1. Use the surface-scraping method to scrape the Pishu and Weishu acupoints from top to bottom.

2. Use the surface-scraping method to scrape the Zusanli and Yinlingquan acupoints of the lower limbs from top to bottom.

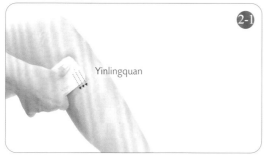

Yinlingquan

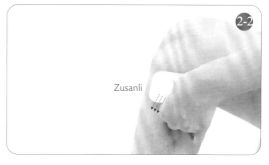

Zusanli

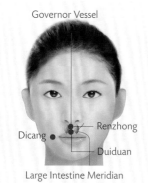

Governor Vessel

Dicang

Renzhong

Duiduan

Large Intestine Meridian

Dark Red Upper Lip

The Large Intestine Meridian and the Governor Vessel run through the upper lip, which is the holographic acupoint area of the bladder, uterus, ovaries, and prostate. Therefore, a dark red upper lip is not only due to the decline in the spleen's transportation and transformation functions, but also stagnated heat in the large intestine and inflammation of the urinary and reproductive organs. Symptoms are more common in people with Bladder Meridian damp heat or ovarian disease.

Facial Beauty *Gua Sha*

1. Clean the facial skin and lips. After applying facial *gua sha* cream, scrape the skin of the upper lip first. Use the pushing and scraping method to scrape the upper lip from the Renzhong acupoint to the Duiduan acupoint, and then push and scrape from the Renzhong and Duiduan acupoints outwards to the Dicang acupoint at the corner of the mouth. Push and scrape Dicang acupoint from bottom to top outwards 5 times. Then flat-press and knead each point 5 times.

   2. Scrape the red part of the upper lip. Place the scraper flat on the lip lines, and use the pushing and scraping method to scrape from the Duiduan acupoint at the tip of the middle of the upper lip to the outside along the upper lip lines to the corner of the mouth. Scrape 5 times. Flat-press and knead the Dicang acupoint 5 times with an outward and upward lifting force. The specific scraping method is the same as that of the upper lip when it is pale and bluish.

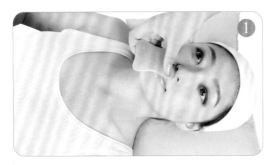

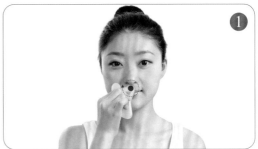

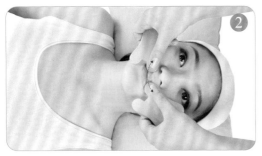

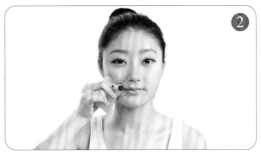

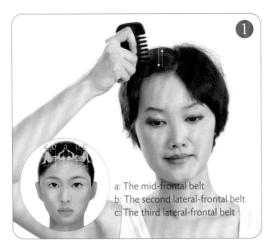

a: The mid-frontal belt
b: The second lateral-frontal belt
c: The third lateral-frontal belt

Consolidating *Gua Sha* on the Head, Hands, and Feet

1. Use the sharp-edge scraping method to scrape the mid-frontal belt, the second lateral-frontal belt and the third lateral-frontal belt on both sides of the head.

   2. Use the pushing and scraping method to scrape the stomach area, large intestine area on the hands and feet, and the gonad area on both sides of the heel.

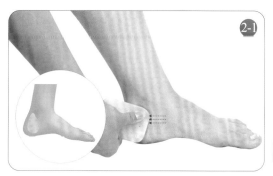

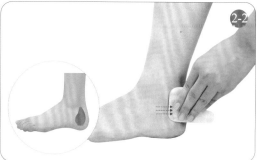

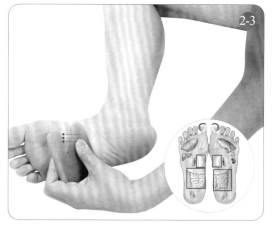

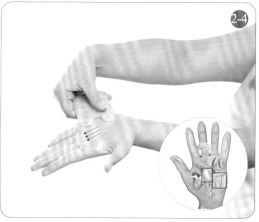

Whole-Body *Gua Sha* and Conditioning

1. Scrape the corresponding area of spleen and stomach on the spine. ① Use the surface-scraping method to scrape the Governor Vessel at the 8th to 12th thoracic vertebrae on the back from top to bottom. ② Use the dual-angle method to scrape the Jiaji acupoints from top to bottom on both sides of the same horizontal section of the Governor Vessel. ③ Then, use the surface-scraping method to scrape the 3-cun wide area on both sides of the Governor Vessel from top to bottom. Focus on the Dazhui, Pishu, Weishu, and

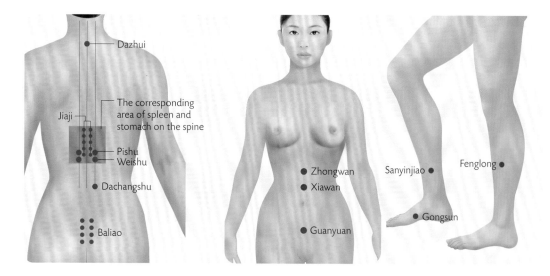

Dachangshu acupoints. For patients with gynecological diseases, scrape the Baliao acupoints too.

2. Use the surface-scraping method to scrape the Zhongwan, Xiawan, and Guanyuan acupoints on the abdomen from top to bottom.

3. Use the surface-scraping method to scrape the Quchi and Hegu acupoints on the upper limbs, Fenglong, Gongsun, and Sanyinjiao acupoints on the lower limbs, from top to bottom.

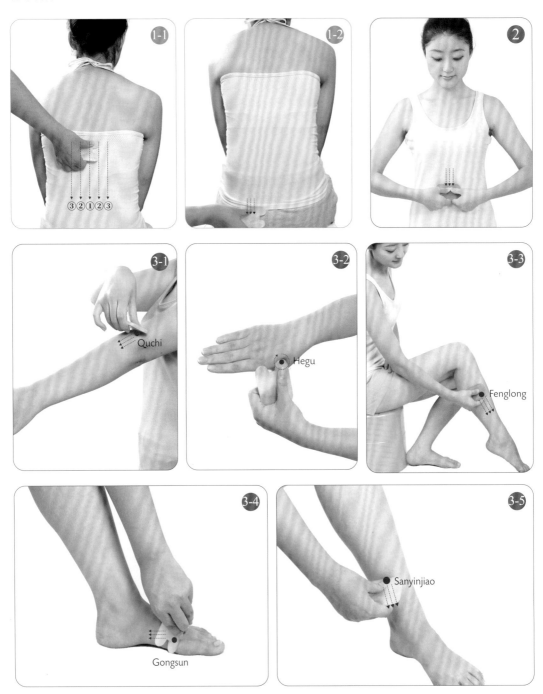

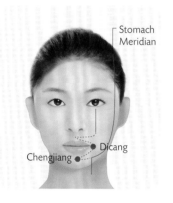

Stomach
Meridian

Dicang

Chengjiang

Crimson Lower Lip

A crimson lower lip is a sign of stomach heat, inflamed
stomach fire, insufficient stomach *yin*, and stomach
inflammation. If the symptoms are accompanied by
acidity, dull stomachache, dry mouth, thirst, bad breath,
and compulsive hunger, you should also be on the lookout
for gastric ulcers.

Facial Beauty *Gua Sha*

1. Clean the facial skin and lips. After applying facial *gua
sha* cream, scrape the skin of the lower lip first. Use the pushing and scraping method to
scrape from the Chengjiang acupoint on the lower jaw outward to the Dicang acupoint at
the corner of the mouth, and scrape the Dicang acupoint from bottom to top outwards.
Scrape 5 times each. Then flat-press and knead each point 5 times.

2. Scrape the red part of the lower lip. Place the scraper flat on the lip lines, and use
the pushing and scraping method to scrape from the middle of the lips outwards to the
corner of the mouth 5 times. Flat-press and knead the Dicang acupoint 5 times with an
upward and outward lifting force. This specific scraping method is the same as that for a
pale lower lip.

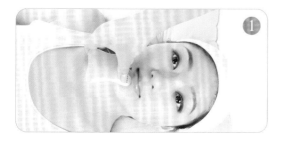

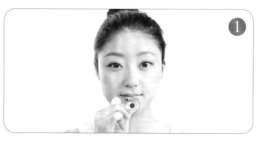

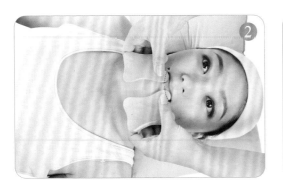
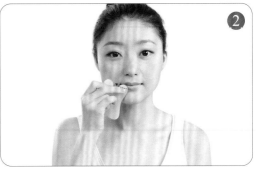

Consolidating *Gua Sha* on the Head, Hands, and Feet

1. Use the sharp-edge scraping method to scrape the second lateral-frontal belt on both sides of the head.

2. Scrape stomach area on the hands and feet with the pushing and scraping method.

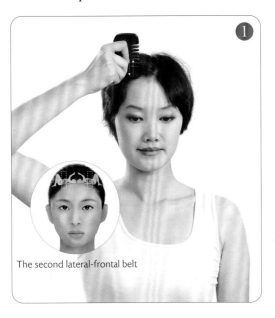

The second lateral-frontal belt

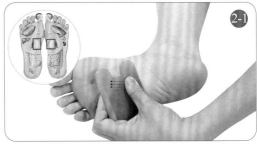

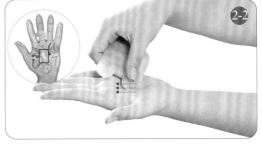

Whole-Body *Gua Sha* and Conditioning

1. Scrape the spine area corresponding to the spleen and stomach. ① Use the surface-scraping method to scrape the Governor Vessel at the 8th to 12th thoracic vertebrae on the back from top to bottom. ② Use the dual-angle scraping method to scrape the Jiaji acupoints from top to bottom on both sides of the same horizontal section of the Governor Vessel. ③ Then, use the surface-scraping method to scrape the 3-cun wide area on both sides of the Governor Vessel from top to bottom. Focus on the Dazhui, Ganshu, Danshu, Pishu, and Weishu acupoints.

2. Use the surface-scraping method to scrape the Shangwan and Zhongwan acupoints on the abdomen from top to bottom.

3. Use the surface-scraping method to scrape the Quchi and Hegu acupoints on upper limbs, and Fenglong and Gongsun acupoints on lower limbs, from top to bottom.

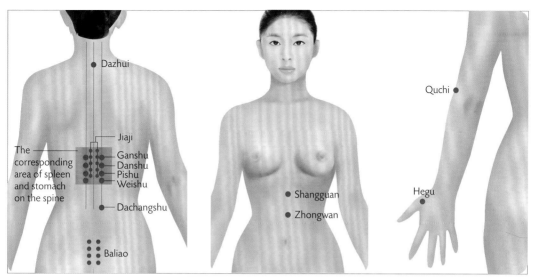

Dazhui

Jiaji

The corresponding area of spleen and stomach on the spine

Ganshu
Danshu
Pishu
Weishu

Dachangshu

Baliao

Shangguan

Zhongwan

Quchi

Hegu

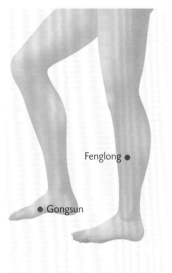

Fenglong

Gongsun

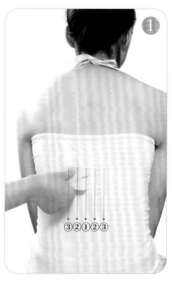

③②①②③

①

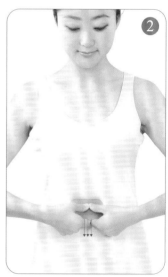

②

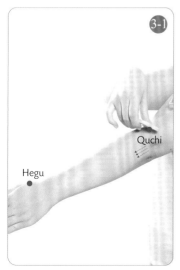

Quchi

Hegu

3-1

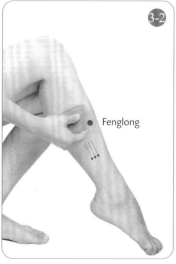

Fenglong

3-2

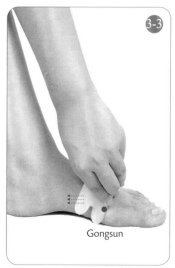

Gongsun

3-3

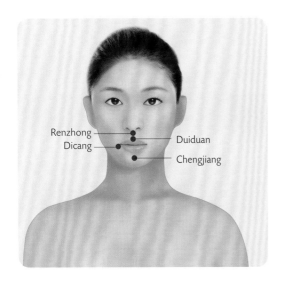

Changes in the Color of the Whole Lip

Bright red lips indicate fever and respiratory infection. Lips turning bluish indicates heart-blood stasis, heart-*yang* deficiency, or drug or food poisoning. Pale lips indicate malnutrition, anemia, hypothermia, and cold hands and feet. Black or dark lips suggest spleen and stomach deficiency-cold and problems with the digestive system. Dark spots appearing on the lips suggest a decline in renal function.

Facial Beauty *Gua Sha*

1. Clean the facial skin and lips. After applying facial *gua sha* cream, scrape the skin of the upper lip first. Use the pushing and scraping method to scrape the upper lip from the Renzhong acupoint to the Duiduan acupoint, and then push and scrape from the Renzhong and Duiduan acupoints outwards to the Dicang acupoint at the corner of the mouth. Push and scrape the Dicang acupoint from bottom outwards to the top 5 times. Then use flat-pressing and kneading to massage each point 5 times.

   2. Scrape the red part of the upper lip. Place the scraper flat on the lip lines. Use the pushing and scraping method to scrape from the Duiduan acupoint to the outside along the upper lip lines to the corner of the mouth, and scrape 5 times.

   3. Scrape the skin of the lower lip. Use the pushing and scraping method to scrape from the Chengjiang acupoint on the lower jaw outwards to the Dicang acupoint at the corner of the mouth, and scrape the Dicang acupoint from the bottom outwards to the top, 5 times each. Then flat-press and knead each point 5 times.

   4. Scrape the red part of the lower lip. Place the scraper flat on the lip lines. Use the pushing and scraping method to scrape from the middle of the lips outwards to the corner of the mouth, and scrape 5 times. Flat-press and knead the Dicang acupoint 5 times with an upward and outward lifting force.

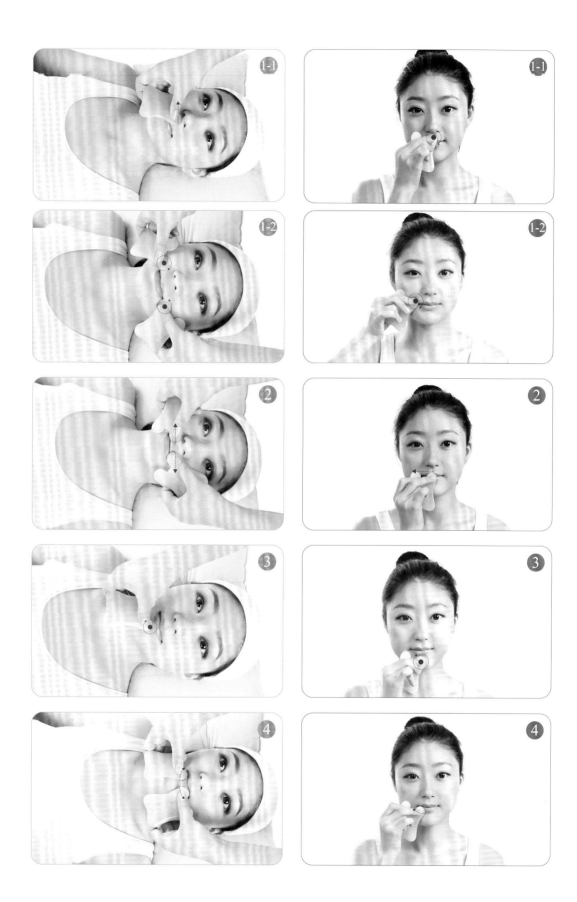

Consolidating *Gua Sha* on the Hands and Feet

Gua sha treatment according to the changes of lip color:

Bright red lips	Use the surface-scraping method to scrape the holographic areas of the lung and spleen on the hands and feet.
Bluish lips	Use the surface-scraping method to scrape the holographic areas of the heart and lung on the hands and feet.
Pale lips	Use the surface-scraping method to scrape the holographic areas of the spleen and kidney on the hands and feet.
Dark lips	Use the surface-scraping method to scrape the holographic areas of the spleen, kidney, and gonad on the hands and feet.

1. Scrape the holographic area of the lung on the hands and feet.
2. Scrape the holographic area of the spleen on the hands and feet.
3. Scrape the holographic area of the heart on the hands and feet.
4. Scrape the holographic area of the kidney on the hands and feet.
5. Scrape the holographic area of the gonad on the hands and feet.

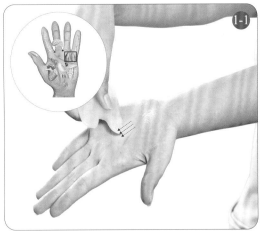
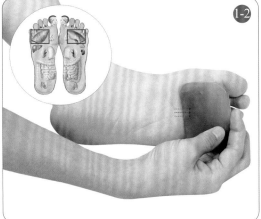
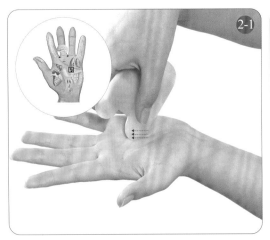
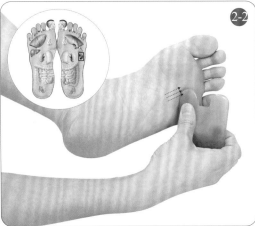

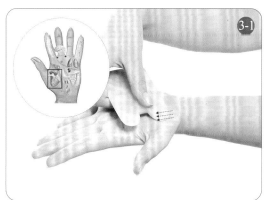

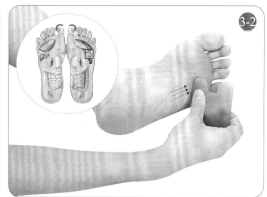

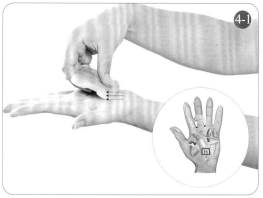

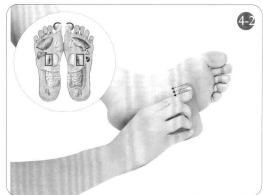

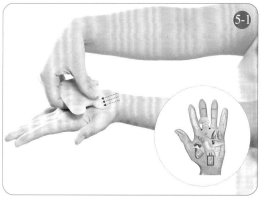

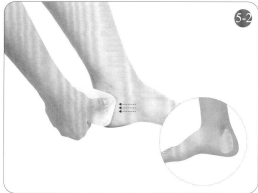

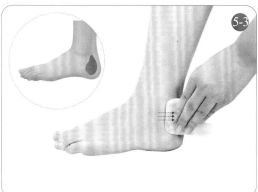

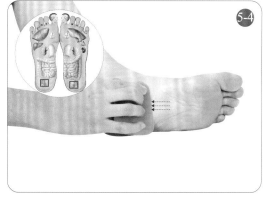

Whole-Body *Gua Sha* and Conditioning

Gua sha treatment according to the changes of lip color:

Bright red lips	Use the surface-scraping method and dual-angle scraping method to scrape the corresponding areas of lung and stomach on the spine from top to bottom, focusing on the Feishu and Weishu acupoints.
Bluish lips	Use the surface-scraping method and dual-angle scraping method to scrape the corresponding area of the heart and lung on the spine from top to bottom, focusing on the Danzhong, Xinshu, and Feishu acupoints.
Pale lips	Use the surface-scraping method to scrape the Pishu, Weishu, and Shenshu acupoints from top to bottom.
Dark lips	Use the surface-scraping method to scrape the Pishu, Weishu, Shenshu, and Baliao acupoints from top to bottom.

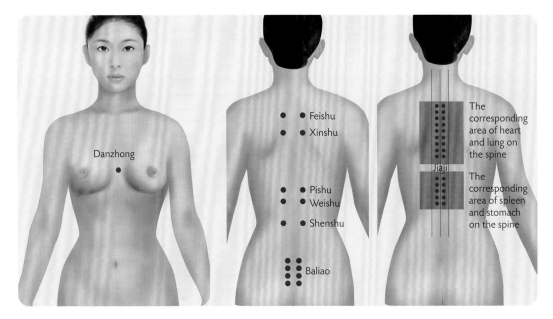

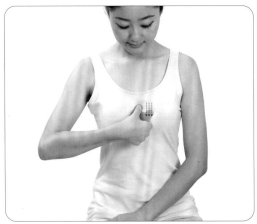
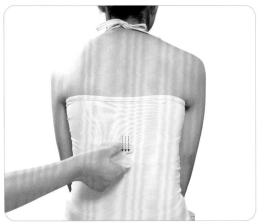

Diet Therapy and Skin Care

If your lips are particularly dry and prone to peeling, do not wet them with saliva, because when it evaporates, it will take away moisture and make your lips drier. Food can be used to condition your body and make your lips bright and moist.

If you suffer from cracked lips, never tear the soft skin with your fingers. Instead, apply a wrung hot towel (not too hot) to the lips first. Remove it after 3 to 5 minutes, then use a soft toothbrush to remove the dead skin from the lips, and gently press the towel on the lips to absorb excess moisture. Then, apply honey or a good quality lip balm that contains ingredients like vitamin E, as thick as possible. Then apply plastic wrap and leave it on for 10 to 15 minutes.

Food Therapy Recipes

• White fungus soup: Take 30 grams of white fungus and wash it. Put it in a clay pot, add water, and stew until cooked. Add rock sugar to taste. Consume twice a day to nourish *yin* and moisten the lungs, relieve coughing, lower blood pressure, and lower fat. Do not take this soup if you have a wind-cold cough or cold.

• Duck soup: Cut the meat from 1 duck, and stew until cooked. After adding seasoning, eat the meat and drink the soup. Taken twice a day. It clears heat, nourishes *yin*, increases body fluids, and moisturizes the skin. Do not consume if you have deficiency-cold or a loss of appetite due to cold, or if you have cold abdominal pain, diarrhea, low back pain, or dysmenorrhea.

• Honey-brewed white pear: Take 1 large white pear, remove the pit, add 50 grams of honey, steam, and eat. Consume twice a day for several days. It works for symptoms such as chapped lips, a dry throat, hot sensation in hands and feet, a dry cough, a chronic cough, and phlegm.

Homemade Lip Masks

• Honey lip mask: Mix 1 spoonful of honey, 1 spoonful of milk, and 1 spoonful of cereal solution, and stir well. Apply a cotton swab dipped in the above solution to your lips and wash off after 20 minutes. The rest can be kept in the refrigerator and used several times. After applying it continuously for a week, your lips will be visibly shinier.

• Yogurt and honey lip mask: Mix leftover yogurt with 1 to 2 drops of honey and stir. Then use a cotton swab dipped in some of the mixture to coat the lips evenly. Apply plastic wrap to the lips and leave for around 15 minutes before washing off with water.

• Olive oil lip mask: Pour some olive oil and honey into container with 2 drops of vitamin E solution (taken from a capsule), and mix well. Brush a thick coating onto the lips. Wipe clean after 15 minutes. This method will make your lips red and shiny, especially in dry fall and winter, and in windy weather.

Location of the Acupoints

Acupoints can be located using the length and width of a person's finger. Please refer to the following for measuring "cun."

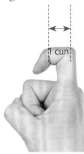 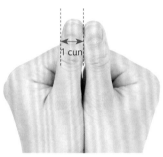 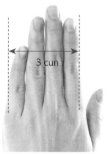

Use middle finger length: The distance between the two inner ends of two cross striation when the middle finger is placed on the body for location of acupoint is 1 cun. This placement method can be used on the lower back and the four limbs.

Use thumb length: The lateral width of the interphalangeal joint of the thumb is taken to be 1 cun. This placement method is commonly used on the four limbs.

Use four fingers closed together: With the index finger, middle finger, ring finger, and small finger of the patient stretched straight and closed, measure at the level of the large knuckle (the second joint) of the middle finger. The width of the four fingers is 3 cun.

Acupoint	Location	Code
Anmian	At the midpoint of the line connecting the Yifeng and Fengchi acupoints.	/
Baihui	On the head, 5 cun superior to the anterior hairline, on the anterior midline.	GV 20
Baliao	There are eight Baliao points in total, four on each side of the sacral spine. These are the upper, secondary, middle and lower Baliao points. They are located respectively in the first, second, third and fourth posterior sacral foramina (opening between vertebrae).	BL 31–34
Benshen	On the head, 0.5 cun superior to the anterior hairline, 3 cun lateral to the anterior midline.	GB 13
Chengjiang	On the face, in the depression in the center of the mentolabial sulcus.	CV 24
Chengqi	On both sides of the face, between the eyeball and the infraorbital margin, directly inferior to the pupil.	ST 1
Chize	On the anterior aspect of both elbows, at the cubital crease, in the depression lateral to the biceps brachii tendon.	LU 5
Cuanzhu	On both sides of the head, in the depression at the medial end of the eyebrow.	BL 2
Dabao	In the lateral thoracic region, in the sixth intercostal space, on the midaxillary line.	SP 21
Dachangshu	In the lumbar region, at the same level as the inferior border of the spinous border of the fourth lumbar vertebra (L 4), 1.5 cun to the posterior midline.	BL 25
Danshu	On both sides of the upper back region, at the same level as the inferior border of the spinous process of the tenth thoracic vertebra (T 10), 1.5 cun lateral to the posterior midline.	BL 19

Acupoint	Location	Code
Danzhong	In the anterior thoracic region, at the same level as the fourth intercostal space, on the anterior midline.	CV 17
Daying	On the face, anterior to the angle of the mandible, in the depression anterior to the masseter attachment, over the facial artery.	ST 5
Dazhu	On both sides of the upper back region, at the same level as the inferior border of the spinous process of the first thoracic vertebra (T 1), 1.5 cun lateral to the posterior midline.	BL 11
Dazhui	In the posterior region of the neck, in the depression inferior to the spinous process of the seventh cervical vertebra, on the posterior midline.	GV 14
Dicang	On the face, 0.4 cun lateral to the angle of the mouth.	ST 4
Duiduan	At the midpoint of the tubercle of the upper lip.	GV 27
Feishu	In the upper back region, at the same level as the inferior border of the spinous process of the third thoracic vertebra, 1.5 cun lateral to the posterior midline.	BL 13
Fengchi	In the posterior region of both sides of the neck, inferior to the occipital bone, in the depression between the origins of the sternocleidomastoid and the trapezius muscles.	GB 20
Fenglong	On the anterolateral aspect of both legs, at the lateral border of the tibialis anterior muscle, 8 cun superior to the prominence of the external malleolus.	ST 40
Ganshu	On both sides of the upper back region, at the same level as the inferior border of the spinous process of the ninth thoracic vertebra, 1.5 cun lateral to the posterior midline.	BL 18
Gaohuang	On both sides of the upper back region, at the same level as the inferior border of the spinous process of the fourth thoracic vertebra (T 4), 3 cun lateral to the posterior midline.	BL 43
Geshu	On both sides of the upper back region, at the same level as the inferior border of the spinous process of the seventh thoracic vertebra (T 7), 1.5 cun lateral to the posterior midline.	BL 17
Gongsun	On the medial aspect of both feet, anteroinferior to the base of the first metatarsal bone, at the border between the red and white flesh.	SP 4
Guanyuan	On the lower abdomen, 3 cun inferior to the center of the umbilicus, on the anterior midline.	CV 4
Guilai	On the lower abdomen, 4 cun inferior to the center of the umbilicus, 2 cun lateral to the anterior midline.	ST 29
Hegu	On the dorsum of both hands, radial to the midpoint of the second metacarpal bone.	LI 4
Hunmen	In the upper back region, at the same level as the inferior border of the spinous process of the ninth thoracic vertebra (T 9), 3 cun lateral to the posterior midline.	BL 47
Jiache	On both sides of the face, one finger breadth (middle finger) anterosuperior to the angle of the mandible.	ST 6
Jiaji	On the spine area, on both sides of the spinous process from the first thoracic vertebra to the fifth lumbar vertebra, 0.5 cun lateral to the middle line of the back, there are seventeen points on each side.	EX-B 2
Jianjing	At the midpoint of the line connecting the spinous process of the seventh cervical vertebra with the lateral end of both acromia.	GB 21
Jianli	On the upper abdomen, 3 cun superior to the center of the umbilicus, on the anterior midline.	CV 11
Jianliao	On both shoulder girdles, in the depression between the acromial angle and the greater tubercle of the humerus.	TE 14

Acupoint	Location	Code
Jianzhen	On both shoulder girdles, posteroinferior to the shoulder joint, 1 cun superior to the posterior axillary fold.	SI 9
Jiexi	On the anterior aspect of both ankles, in the depression at the center of the front surface of the ankle joint, between the tendons of extensor hallucis longus and extensor digitorum longus.	ST 41
Jingming	On both sides of the face, in the depression between the superomedial parts of the inner canthus of the eye and the medial wall of the orbit.	BL 1
Jinsuo	In the upper back region, in the depression inferior to the spinous process of the ninth thoracic vertebra (T 9), on the posterior midline.	GV 8
Juegu (or Xuanzhong)	On the fibular aspect of the leg, anterior to the fibula, 3 cun proximal to the prominence of the lateral malleolus.	GB 39
Juque	On the upper abdomen, 6 cun superior to the center of the umbilicus, on the anterior midline.	CV 14
Kouheliao	Directly below the nostril, at the level of 1/3 of the nasolabial groove.	LI 19
Lianquan	In the anterior region of the neck, superior to the thyroid cartilage, in the depression superior to the hyoid bone, on the anterior midline.	CV 23
Lieque	On the radial aspect of both forearms, between the tendons of the abductor pollicis longus and the extensor pollicis brevis muscles, in the groove for the abductor pollicis longus tendon, 1.5 cun superior to the palmar wrist crease.	LU 7
Ligou	On the anteromedial aspect of both legs, at the center of the medial border (surface) of the tibia, 5 cun proximal to the prominence of the medial malleolus.	LR 5
Meichong	Push upward from Cuanzhu point (BL 2), 0.5 cun within the hairline, where pain will be felt on pressure.	BL 3
Mingmen	In the lumbar region, in the depression inferior to the spinous process of the second lumbar vertebra (L 2), on the posterior midline.	GV 4
Neiguan	On the anterior aspect of both forearms, between the tendons of the palmaris longus and the flexor carpi radialis, 2 cun proximal to the palmar wrist crease.	PC 6
Neixiyan	On both knees and in the center of the depression of the patellar ligament.	EX-LE 4
Pangguangshu	In the sacral region, at the same level as the second posterior sacral foramen, and 1.5 cun lateral to the median sacral crest.	BL 28
Pishu	On both sides of the upper back region, at the same level as the inferior border of the spinous process of the 11th thoracic vertebra (T 11), 1.5 cun lateral to the posterior midline.	BL 20
Qihai	On the lower abdomen, 1.5 cun directly below the umbilicus, on the anterior midline.	CV 6
Qimen	On both sides of the anterior thoracic region, in the sixth intercostal space, 4 cun lateral to the anterior midline.	LR 14
Qiuxu	On the anterolateral aspect of both ankles, in the depression lateral to the extensor digitorum longus tendon, anterior and distal to the lateral malleolus.	GB 40
Qixue	On the lower abdomen, 4 cun inferior to the center of the umbilicus, 0.5 cun lateral to the anterior midline.	KI 13
Quanliao	On the face, inferior to the zygomatic bone, in the depression directly inferior to the outer canthus of the eye.	SI 18
Quchi	On the lateral aspect of both elbows, at the midpoint of the line connecting Chize point (LU 5) with the lateral epicondyle of the humerus.	LI 11
Ququan	On the medial aspect of both knees, in the depression medial to the tendons of the semitendinosus and the semimembranosus muscles, at the medial end of the popliteal crease.	LR 8

Acupoint	Location	Code
Quze	On the anterior aspect of both elbows, at the cubital crease, in the depression medial to the biceps brachii tendon.	PC 3
Renzhong	On the face, at the upper 1/3 of the philtrum. Also called Shuigou.	GV 26
Riyue	In the anterior thoracic region, in the seventh intercostal space, 4 cun lateral to the anterior midline.	GB 24
Sanjiaoshu	On both sides of the lumbar region, at the same level as the inferior border of the spinous process of the first lumbar vertebra (L 1), 1.5 cun lateral to the posterior midline.	BL 22
Sanyinjiao	On the tibial aspect of both legs, posterior to the medial border of the tibia, 3 cun superior to the prominence of the medial malleolus.	SP 6
Shangguan	On the head, in the depression superior to the midpoint of the zygomatic arch.	GB 3
Shangjuxu	On the anterior aspect of both legs, on the line connecting Dubi point (ST 35) with Jiexi point (ST 41), 6 cun inferior to Dubi point (ST 35).	ST 37
Shangyingxiang	On the face, at the junction between the alar cartilages and turbinate, and close to the upper edge of the nasolabial groove.	EX-HN 8
Shaohai	On the anteromedial aspect of both elbows, just anterior to the medial epicondyle of the humerus, at the same level as the cubital crease.	HT 3
Shenmen	On the anteromedial aspect of both wrists, radial to the flexor carpi ulnaris tendon, on the palmar wrist crease.	HT 7
Shenshu	On both sides of the lumbar region, at the same level as the inferior border of the spinous process of the second lumbar vertebra (L 2), 1.5 cun lateral to the posterior midline.	BL 23
Shentang	In the upper back region, at the same level as the inferior border of the spinous process of the fifth thoracic vertebra (T 5), 3 cun lateral to the posterior midline.	BL 44
Shenting	On the head, 0.5 cun superior to the anterior hairline, on the anterior midline.	GV 24
Shuifen	On the upper abdomen, 1 cun superior to the center of the umbilicus, on the anterior midline.	CV 9
Shuiquan	On the medial aspect of both feet, 1 cun inferior to Taixi (KI 3), in the depression of the medial side of the calcaneal tuberosity.	KI 5
Sibai	On both sides of the face, in the infraorbital foramen.	ST 2
Sizhukong	On the face, in the depression at the lateral end of the eyebrows.	TE 23
Suliao	On the face, at the tip of the nose.	GV 25
Taichong	On the dorsum of both feet, between the first and second metatarsal bones, in the depression distal to the junction of the bases of the two bones, over the dorsalis pedis artery.	LR 3
Taixi	On the posteromedial aspect of both ankles, in the depression between the prominence of the medial malleolus and the calcaneal tendon.	KI 3
Taiyang	On the temporal of both sides of the face, in the depression lateral to the outer end of eyebrows.	EX-HN 5
Taiyuan	On the anterolateral aspect of both wrists, between the radial styloid process and the scaphoid bone, in the depression ulnar to the abductor pollicis longus tendon.	LU 9
Tianzhu	In the posterior region of both sides of the neck, at the same level as the superior border of the spinous process of the second cervical vertebra (C 2), in the depression lateral to the trapezius muscle.	BL 10
Tianzong	In the scapular region of both sides of the body, in the depression between the upper 1/3 and lower 2/3 of the line connecting the inferior border of spine of the scapula with the inferior angle of the scapula.	SI 11

Acupoint	Location	Code
Tinggong	On both sides of the face, in the depression between the anterior border of the center of the tragus and the posterior border of the condylar process of the mandible.	SI 19
Tongli	On the anteromedial aspect of both forearms, radial to the flexor carpi ulnaris tendon, 1 cun proximal to the palmar wrist crease.	HT 5
Tongziliao	On the face, in the depression 0.5 cun lateral to the outer canthus of the eyes.	GB 1
Toulinqi	On the head, 0.5 cun superior to the anterior hairline, midpoint of eyebrows, directly superior to the center of the pupil.	GB 15
Touwei	On both sides of the head, 0.5 cun directly superior to the anterior hairline at the corner of the forehead, 4.5 cun lateral to the anterior midline.	ST 8
Waiguan	On the posterior aspect of both forearms, 2 cun proximal to the dorsal wrist crease, the midpoint of the interosseous space between the radius and the ulna.	TE 5
Waiqiu	On the fibular aspect of the leg, anterior to the fibula, 7 cun proximal to the prominence of the lateral malleolus.	GB 36
Waixiyan (or Dubi)	On the anterior aspect of both knees, in the depression lateral to the patellar ligament.	ST 35
Weishu	On both sides of the upper back region, at the same level as the inferior border of the spinous process of the 12th thoracic vertebra (T 12), 1.5 cun lateral to the posterior midline.	BL 21
Weiyang	On the posterolateral aspect of both knees, just medial to the biceps femoris tendon in the popliteal crease.	BL 39
Weizhong	On the posterior aspect of both knees, at the midpoint of the popliteal crease.	BL 40
Xiaguan	On both sides of the face, in the depression between the midpoint of the inferior border of the zygomatic arch and the mandibular notch.	ST 7
Xiaochangshu	On both sides of the sacral region, at the same level as the first posterior sacral foramen, and 1.5 cun lateral to the median sacral crest.	BL 27
Xiaohai	On the posteromedial aspect of both elbows, in the depression between the olecranon and the medial epicondyle of the humerus bone.	SI 8
Xiawan	On the upper abdomen, 2 cun superior to the center of the umbilicus, on the anterior midline.	CV 10
Xiaxi	On the dorsum of both feet, between the fourth and fifth toes, proximal to the web margin, at the border between the red and white flesh.	GB 43
Xinshu	On both sides of the upper back region, at the same level as the inferior border of the spinous process of the fifth thoracic vertebra (T 5), 1.5 cun lateral to the posterior midline.	BL 15
Xiyangguan	On the lateral aspect of the knee, in the depression between the biceps femoris tendon and the iliotibial band.	GB 33
Xuehai	On the anteromedial aspect of both thighs, on the bulge of the vastus medialis muscle, 2 cun superior to the medial end of the base of the patella.	SP 10
Yamen	In the posterior region of the neck, in the depression inferior to the spinous process of the second cervical vertebra (C 2), on the posterior midline.	GV 15
Yangbai	On the head, 1 cun superior to the eyebrows, directly superior to the center of the pupil.	GB 14
Yanggang	In the upper back region, at the same level as the inferior border of the spinous process of the tenth thoracic vertebra (T 10), 3 cun lateral to the posterior midline.	BL 48
Yanglingquan	On the fibular aspect of both legs, in the depression anterior and distal to the head of the fibula.	GB 34
Yaoshu	In the sacral region, at the sacral hiatus, on the posterior midline.	GV 2

Acupoint	Location	Code
Yaoyangguan	In the lumbar region, in the depression inferior to the spinous process of the fourth lumbar vertebra (L 4), on the posterior midline.	GV 3
Yifeng	In the anterior region of the neck, posterior to the ear lobe on both sides, in the depression anterior to the inferior end of the mastoid process.	TE 17
Yin'gu	On the posterior aspect of the knees, at the exterior border of the semitendinosus tendon, on the popliteal fossa.	KI 10
Yingxiang	On both sides of the face, in the nasolabial sulcus, at the same level as the midpoint of the lateral border of the ala of the nose.	LI 20
Yinjiao	At the junction of the frenulum of the upper lip with the upper gum.	GV 28
Yinlingquan	On the tibial aspect of both legs, in the depression between the inferior border of the medial condyle of the tibia and the medial border of the tibia.	SP 9
Yintang	On the forehead, in the depression of the middle of the two eyebrows' medial end.	GV 29
Yinxi	On the anteromedial aspect of the forearms, radial to the flexor carpi ulnaris tendon, 0.5 cun proximal to the palmar wrist crease.	HT 6
Yishu	On the spine area, on the horizontal line of the lower edge of the eighth thoracic spinous process, 1.5 cun lateral to the middle line of the back.	EX-B 3
Yongquan	In the sole of both feet, in the deepest depression when the foot is in plantar flexion.	KI 1
Yunmen	On both sides of the anterior thoracic region, in the depression of the infraclavicular fossa, medial to the coracoid process of the scapula, 6 cun lateral to the anterior median line.	LU 2
Yuyao	On both sides of the forehead, straight superior to the pupils, in the eyebrow.	EX-HN 4
Zhangmen	On both sides of the lateral abdomen, inferior to the free extremity of the 11th rib.	LR 13
Zhigou	On the posterior aspect of the forearms, the midpoint of the interosseous space between the radius and the ulna, 3 cun proximal to the dorsal wrist crease.	TE 6
Zhishi	On both sides of the lumbar region, at the same level as the inferior border of the spinous process of the second lumbar vertebra (L 2), 3 cun lateral to the posterior midline.	BL 52
Zhiyang	In the upper back region, in the depression inferior to the spinous process of the seventh thoracic vertebra (T 7), on the posterior midline.	GV 9
Zhizheng	On the posteromedial aspect of the forearms, between the medial border of the ulnar bone and the flexor carpi ulnaris muscle, 5 cun proximal to the dorsal-wrist crease.	SI 7
Zhongfu	On both sides of the anterior thoracic region, at the same level as the first intercostal space, lateral to the infraclavicular fossa, 6 cun lateral to the anterior median line.	LU 1
Zhongshu	In the upper back region, in the depression inferior to the spinous process of the tenth thoracic vertebra (T 10), on the posterior midline.	GV 7
Zhongwan	On the upper abdomen, 4 cun superior to the center of the umbilicus, on the anterior midline.	CV 12
Zhongzhu	On the dorsum of the hands, between the fourth and fifth metacarpal bones, in the depression proximal to the fourth metacarpophalangeal joint.	TE 3
Zhongzhu	On the lower abdomen, 1 cun inferior to the umbilicus, 0.5 cun lateral to the anterior midline.	KI 15
Zusanli	On the anterior aspect of both legs, on the line connecting Dubi point (ST 35) and Jiexi point (ST 41), 3 cun inferior to Dubi point (ST 35).	ST 36